SPRINGHOUSE

NOTES™

ONCOLOGIC NURSING

JoAnn Huang Eriksson, RN, MS

Ms. Eriksson, the author of this book, is an Associate Professor of Nursing at Rush University, Chicago, Illinois. She is also a Practitioner/Teacher for the Department of Operating Rooms and Surgical Nursing and a Clinical Nurse Specialist for the Department of Gynecologic Oncology at Rush Presbyterian, St. Luke's Medical Center, Chicago. Ms. Eriksson earned her BSN and MSN from Rush University, Chicago. She is a member of the Oncology Nursing Society, Chicago Chapter of the Oncology Nursing Society, Society of Gynecologic Nurse Oncologists, American Nurses' Association, American Nurses' Association Council of Clinical Specialists, Illinois Nurses' Association, and Sigma Theta Tau.

Patricia Darlene Lee, RN, MN, ONS

Ms. Lee, the reviewer of this book, is an Assistant Professor of Nursing at McNeese State University, Lake Charles, Louisiana. She is also a practicing Oncology Nurse Specialist. Ms. Lee earned her BSN from the University of Southwest Louisiana and her MN from Louisiana State University Medical Center. She is currently in the dissertation stage of her PhD at Texas Women's University. Ms. Lee is a member of the American Nurses' Association and the Association of Operating Room Nurses.

Springhouse Corporation
Springhouse, Pennsylvania

D1531621

Staff

Executive Director, Editorial
Stanley Loeb

Executive Director, Creative Services
Jean Robinson

Director of Trade and Textbooks
Minnie B. Rose, RN, BSN, MEd

Art Director
John Hubbard

Consultant
Maryann Foley, RN, BSN

Acquisitions Editor
Donna L. Hilton, RN, BSN, CEN

Editors
Kevin Law (manager), Judd Howard

Copy Editors
David Prout (manager), Diane M. Armento

Designers
Stephanie Peters (associate art director),
Julie Carleton Barlow

Art Production
Robert Perry (manager), Anna Brindisi, Donald
Knauss, Catherine Mace, Robert Wieder

Typography
David Kosten (manager), Diane Paluba (assistant
manager), Joyce Rossi Biletz, Brenda C. Mayer,
Robin Rantz, Brent Rinedoller, Valerie L. Rosenberger

Manufacturing
Deborah Meiris (manager), T.A. Landis,
Jennifer Suter

Production Coordination
Aline S. Miller (manager), Maura C. Murphy

nizations that have been granted a license by CCC, a separate system of payment has been arranged. The fee code for users of the Transactional Reporting Service is 0874342031/90 $00.00 + $.75.
Printed in the United States of America.

SN11-010789

Library of Congress Cataloging-in-Publication Data
Eriksson, JoAnn Huang.
  Oncologic nursing / JoAnn Huang Eriksson:
[reviewed by] Patricia Darlene Lee.
  p. cm. — (Springhouse notes)
  Includes bibliographies and index.
  1. Cancer—Nursing.   I. Lee, Patricia Darlene.
  II. Title.   III. Series.
  [DNLM: 1. Neoplasms—nursing. WY 156 E68o]
RC266.E75 1990
610.73'698—dc20
DNLM/DLC
for Library of Congress   89-6260
ISBN 0-87434-203-1   CIP

Contents

How to Use Springhouse Notes 4

I. Overview of Cancer 5

II. General Principles of Cancer Therapy 12

III. Antineoplastic Agents 25

IV. Nutrition and Cancer 33

V. Nursing Management of Common
Cancer-Related Problems 40

VI. Nursing Management of Patient and
Family Psychosocial Needs 53

VII. Cancer of the Skin 63

VIII. Cancer of the Head, Neck, and Chest 70

IX. Cancer of the GI Tract 80

X. Cancer of the Urinary Tract 100

XI. Cancer of the Reproductive System 109

XII. Cancer of the Hematologic System 134

XIII. Oncologic Emergencies 148

Index 159

How to Use Springhouse Notes

Today, more than ever, nursing students face enormous time pressures. Nursing education has become more sophisticated, increasing the difficulties students have with studying efficiently and keeping pace.

The need for a comprehensive, well-designed series of study aids is great, which is why we've produced Springhouse Notes...to meet that need. Springhouse Notes provide essential course material in outline form, enabling the nursing student to study more effectively, improve understanding, achieve higher test scores, and get better grades.

Key features appear throughout each book, making the information more accessible and easier to remember.
- **Learning Objectives.** These objectives precede each section in the book to help the student evaluate knowledge before and after study.
- **Key Points.** Highlighted in color throughout the book, these points provide a way to quickly review critical information. Key points may include:
—a cardinal sign or symptom of a disorder
—the most current or popular theory about a topic
—a distinguishing characteristic of a disorder
—the most important step of a process
—a critical assessment component
—a crucial nursing intervention
—the most widely used or successful therapy or treatment.
- **Points to Remember.** This information, found at the end of each section, summarizes the section in capsule form.
- **Glossary.** Difficult, frequently used, or sometimes misunderstood terms are defined for the student at the end of each section.

Remember: Springhouse Notes are learning tools designed to *help* you. They are not intended for use as a primary information source. They should never substitute for class attendance, text reading, or classroom note-taking.

This book, *Oncologic Nursing,* applies the general principles of surgery, radiation therapy, and chemotherapy to the major types of cancer. It also addresses important concepts such as nutrition and psychosocial needs of the patient and family. The sections on the major cancers are grouped according to the body system affected and organized according to the nursing process. Specific information on cancer-related problems and emergencies also are approached through the nursing process. The statistical information included reflects a synopsis of current major reference sources. Keep in mind that medical, surgical, and nursing interventions may include more than one option in the progression of care and must be prioritized and adapted to meet the individual patient's needs.

Overview of Cancer

Learning Objectives

After studying this section, the reader should be able to:

- Differentiate between benign and malignant neoplasms.

- Identify three treatment modalities used in cancer therapy.

- Discuss the purpose of cancer staging systems.

- State two events involved in carcinogenesis.

- Identify the four routes of tumor metastasis.

- Discuss how tumor cells may escape destruction by the immune system.

I. Overview of Cancer
A. Introduction
1. Terminology used in oncology
   a. Neoplasm: an autonomous and abnormal growth of tissue
   b. Hyperplasia: abnormal increase in the number of cells in a tissue
   c. Metaplasia: reversible process of one adult cell type replacing another cell type; e.g., during squamous metaplasia, squamous cells replace columnar cells of the endocervix
   d. Dysplasia: changes of adult cell size, shape, and organization
   e. Anaplasia: cellular disorganization characterized by positional or cytologic alterations
2. Cancer affects the life cycle of normal cells
3. In the cancer cell cycle, cells lose the mechanisms that control cell division and growth; e.g., mitosis results in the formation of several new cells rather than the normally expected two new cells
4. Accepted cancer treatment modalities include:
   a Surgery
   b. Radiation therapy
   c. Chemotherapy
   d. Combinations of these three modalities
5. Treatment modalities currently under investigation include:
   a. Biological response modifiers (BRM): using immunotherapeutic agents to augment or simulate natural immune functions in an attempt to alter the relationship between tumor cells and host response
   b. Hyperthermia: artificially elevating body temperature to kill cancer cells
   c. Intraoperative radiation therapy: surgically debulking the tumor and exposing an area for treatment with radiation therapy
   d. Autologous bone marrow rescue: reinfusing harvested bone marrow to replace blood components destroyed by the highly cytotoxic doses of chemotherapeutic agents administered to kill tumor cells
6. Unproven treatment modalities include:
   a. Machines, devices, drugs, and nutritional or psychological regimens
   b. Laetrile
   c. Simonton method of visualization and imagery
   d. Macrobiotic diet
   e. Hoxsey method of using pills to restore the body's chemical balance
   f. Metabolic methods of preventing exposure to toxins and eliminating body wastes
   g. Psychic surgery
7. Cancer treatment settings include:
   a. Ambulatory care settings
   b. Inpatient hospital settings
   c. Home settings

    d. Nursing or convalescent home
    e. Hospice care (both a setting and a concept of care provision)

B. Classification of neoplasms
  1. Biologic classification
    a. Benign: mass of cells that grow slowly; does not metastasize or threaten the host's survival
    b. Malignant: mass of cells that is capable of metastasis and can threaten the host's survival
  2. Histologic classification
    a. Based on the *type of tissue* in which growth originates; e.g., malignant growths originating in the epidermis are called epidermal carcinomas
    b. Based on the *degree of differentiation* of tumor cells (the greater the degree of differentiation, the greater the tumor cell's similarity to the tissue of origin): grade 1 (well differentiated), grade 2 (moderately well differentiated), grade 3 (poorly differentiated), and grade 4 (undifferentiated)
  3. Anatomic classification: staging
    a. Staging is a classification system based on the extent of the disease
    b. A staging system provides standard descriptions of the disease to facilitate communication between health care providers
    c. Of the many existing staging systems, the tumor, node, metastasis (TNM) system is the most frequently used. In this system, T refers to primary tumor; N, to regional lymph node involvement; and M, to metastasis
    d. Cancer type often determines the staging system used. For example, the TNM staging system usually is used in breast cancer, but the International Federation of Gynecologic Oncologists (FIGO) staging system usually is used in ovarian cancer
  4. Neoplastic nomenclature
    a. Benign tumors end with the suffix *-oma* (e.g., cystoma, adenoma), or with the designation *tumor*
    b. Malignant tumors are named according to the germ layer tissue of origin and end with the suffix *-carcinoma* (e.g., adenocarcinoma) or *-sarcoma* (e.g., osteosarcoma)
    c. Carcinomas originate in *endodermal* tissues (which develop into internal structures, such as the stomach and intestines) and *ectodermal* tissues (which develop into external structures, such as the skin)
    d. Sarcomas originate in *mesodermal* tissues, which develop into supporting structures such as bone, muscle, fat, or blood

C. Theories of carcinogenesis
  1. Carcinogenesis is the process by which normal cells transform into tumor cells
  2. Various theories of carcinogenesis are currently under investigation in an attempt to identify factors that promote tumor growth

THE TUMOR, NODE, METASTASIS (TNM) SYSTEM OF CANCER STAGING

MODEL CLASSIFICATION

T0: No evidence of a primary lesion found grossly or microscopically. Evidence of malignant change without microinvasion and without a target lesion identifiable clinically.

T1: A lesion confined to the organ of origin. It is mobile, does not invade adjacent or surrounding structures or tissues, and is often superficial.

T2: A localized lesion characterized by deep extension into adjacent structures or tissues. Invasion is into capsules, ligaments, intrinsic muscle, and adjacent attached structures of similar tissue or function. There is some loss of tumor mobility, but it is not complete; therefore, fixation is not present.

T3: An advanced lesion that is confined to the region rather than to the organ of origin, whether solid or hollow. The critical criterion is fixation, which indicates invasion into a fixed structure or past a boundary. These structures are most often bone and cartilage; but invasion of the extrinsic muscle walls, serosa, and skin are also included. Surrounding detached structures of different anatomy or function are in this category; however, this inclusion can be debated because of the varieties of anatomic stuctures.

T4: A massive lesion extending into another hollow organ causing a fistula, or into another solid organ causing a sinus. Invasions into major nerves, arteries, and veins are placed in this category. Destruction of bone in addition to fixation is an advanced sign.

N0: No evidence of disease in lymph nodes.

N1: Palpable and movable lymph nodes limited to the first station. A distinction between an uninvolved and an involved palpable node needs to be made. This depends on the firmness and roundness of a node and its size, which is generally greater than 1 cm ($\frac{1}{4}$") and often more than 2 cm ($\frac{3}{4}$")—usually up to 3 cm ($1\frac{1}{4}$") in size and solitary.

N2: Firm to hard nodes, palpable and partially movable; they range from 3 to 5 cm ($1\frac{1}{4}$" to 2") in size. Such nodes show microscopic evidence of capsular invasion; clinically, they may be matted together. Nodes can be contralateral or bilateral.

N3: Fixation is complete. Nodes beyond the capsule with complete fixation to bone, to large blood vessels, to skin, or to nerves—usually greater than 6 cm ($2\frac{1}{4}$") in size.

N4: Nodes involved beyond the first station; they are in the second or distant stations. If the first two nodal stations are vertically arranged and both are involved, such double involvement is staged as N4.

NX: Nodes inaccessible to clinical evaluation.

NL: Nodes evaluated by lymphangiography. L− refers to a negative study and L+ to a positive study. An equivocal finding can be referred to as L± if equivocally positive and L∓ if equivocally negative.

N− or N+: Nodes evaluated by microscopic study and designated as a negative or positive depending upon findings.

M0: No evidence of metastases.

M1: Solitary, isolated metastasis confined to one organ or anatomic site.

M2: Multiple metastatic foci confined to one organ system or one anatomic site, e.g., lungs, skeleton, or liver, with no functional to minimal functional impairment of system or site.

M3: Multiple organs involved anatomically, with no or minimial to moderate functional impairment of involved organs.

M4: Multiple organs involved anatomically, with moderate to severe functional impairment of involved organs.

MX: No metastatic workup done.

M: Modified to show viscera involved by letter subscript: pulmonary metastases (M_p), hepatic (M_h), osseous (M_o), skin (M_s), brain (M_b), and so on.

M+: Microscopic evidence of suspected metastases, confirmed by pathologic examination.

*From Rubin, P., ed.: *Clinical Oncology: A Multisiciplinary Approach*, 6th ed. New York: American Cancer Society, 1983.

3. Most of these theories suggest that carcinogenesis involves two or more
    events
    a. Initial event: cell exposure to an initiating factor, such as radiation,
        chemicals, or viruses, that transform and damage the cells; some theories
        propose genetic defects as the initial event
    b. Secondary events: cell exposure to additional factors that promote the
        growth of the transformed cells; exposure may occur shortly after the
        initial event or much later. Drugs, special diets, or other factors may
        reverse effects of the secondary event, but cannot reverse the initial event

D. Invasion and metastasis
1. General information
    a. Invasion refers to disease expansion into surrounding tissue resulting
        from pressure caused by continuous cancer cell division and destruction
        of surrounding tissues by enzymes released from cancer cells
    b. Metastasis refers to dissemination of cancer cells into areas distant from
        the primary tumor
2. Routes of metastasis
    a. Seeding: a primary tumor sloughs off tumor cells into a body cavity,
        such as the peritoneal cavity
    b. Transplantation: tumor cells are transported from one body location to
        another by external means, such as instruments or hands during surgery
    c. Lymphatic spread: tumor cells migrate to distant sites through lymphatic
        channels
    d. Hematogenous spread: tumor cells migrate to distant sites through
        arteries and veins
3. Stages of metastasis
    a. Cells detach from the primary tumor due to lack of cell adhesiveness
    b. Tumor cells invade lymphatic channels or blood vessels
    c. Tumor cells or cell clusters migrate to distant sites
    d. Tumor cells attach to blood vessels of distant organs
    e. Tumor cells invade distant organs through blood vessel walls
    f. Tumor cells grow in organs distant from primary tumor;
        neovascularization resulting from a tumor angiogenesis factor may enable
        tumor growth in distant sites

E. Function of the immune system in cancer
1. The immune system apparently plays a role in regulating the development
    and growth of certain tumors
2. Theories of how tumor cells escape from the immune system include:
    a. Tumor burden is too small to activate the immune system
    b. Tumor burden is too large and overwhelms the immune system

    c. Tumor antigens are too similar to normal antigens to allow recognition as abnormal by the immune system

    d. Tumor cell fibrin coating prevents recognition by the immune system

    e. Antigens shed by tumor cells bind with circulating antibodies and prevent antibodies from reaching the tumor cells

    f. Tumors may produce certain factors which suppress immune system function

3. Immune surveillance theory states that:

    a. Tumor cells express new antigens

    b. The immune system can recognize tumor antigens

    c. The threshold concentration of tumor antigen must be reached to activate the immune system

    d. The immune system of children and elderly persons are not fully functional, which often allows tumor antigens to escape recognition

Points to Remember

Tumor classification is based on cell type and tissue of origin.

Staging systems reflect the extent of cancer and provide some indication of prognosis.

A major factor distinguishing malignant neoplasms from benign neoplasms is malignant neoplasms' ability to invade and metastasize.

An initiating event must occur in order for cancer to develop.

Some theories propose that immune system malfunctions allow cancer to develop.

Glossary

Differentiation—process in which a cell acquires its mature form and function

Histology—microscopic study of cell and tissue structure

Hospice—program of providing palliative care for terminally ill patients and their families; a care-providing concept that also may be an actual physical setting

Neovascularization—development of new blood supply

Tumor angiogenesis factor—agent produced by a tumor that enables the development of a new blood supply

General Principles of Cancer Therapy

Learning Objectives

After studying this section, the reader should be able to:

- Identify the guiding principle in each cancer treatment modality.

- Define possible goals for each treatment modality.

- Identify several types of surgery for cancer.

- Discuss appropriate nursing interventions for a patient undergoing such surgery.

- Identify two types of radiation therapy.

- Describe the safety guidelines for radiation therapy.

- Discuss appropriate nursing interventions for a patient undergoing radiation therapy.

- Describe protective measures the nurse should use when handling and administering antineoplastic agents.

- Discuss appropriate nursing interventions for a patient receiving chemotherapy.

II. General Principles of Cancer Therapy

A. Introduction
1. Decisions on treatment modality are based on:
   a. Cancer location
   b. Histologic cell type
   c. Degree of tumor dissemination
   d. Patient's condition
   e. Goal of treatment
   f. Risk of complications or adverse effects
   g. Patient's desired quality of life
2. Goals of cancer treatment
   a. Cure: eradicate the cancer and promote long-term patient survival
   b. Control: arrest tumor growth
   c. Palliation: alleviate symptoms when disease is beyond control
   d. Prophylaxis: provide treatment when no tumor is detectable but when the patient is known to be at risk for tumor development, spread, or recurrence
3. Types of cancer treatment
   a. Primary: initial treatment given to eradicate disease
   b. Adjuvant: additional treatment given to eliminate microscopic disease and promote cure or improve patient response
   c. Salvage: treatment given to attempt cure after a recurrence

B. Surgery
1. General information
   a. At one time, surgery was the only mode of curative treatment available
   b. Today, surgery is used both alone and in conjunction with chemotherapy, radiation therapy, and immunotherapy
2. Guiding principles for cancer surgery
   a. The patient must understand the possible impairments that can result from surgery
   b. The patient must understand the importance of tumor removal and be told that the surgery will be as radical as necessary to accomplish this
   c. Adequate margins for resection necessitate maximum tumor exposure
   d. Cancer tissue is friable and must be handled delicately; a "no touch" technique minimizes tumor seeding and recurrence
   e. Free cancer cells in the surgical site can cause tumor recurrence; glove and instrument changes and wound irrigation may reduce the risk of local recurrence
   f. Curative procedures involve en bloc resection; blood and lymph vessels are ligated before resection to prevent the escape of cancer cells from the surgical site
3. Goals of surgery
   a. Disease diagnosis
   b. Patient cure

    c. Symptom palliation

    d. Disease prevention

    e. Defect reconstruction and patient rehabilitation

4. Factors affecting a patient's response to cancer surgery
    a. Age
    b. Health status
    c. Nutritional status
    d. Cancer type
    e. Disease stage
    f. Tumor grade
    g. Tumor location
    h. Presence of residual disease (following resection)
5. *Diagnostic surgery*, used to diagnose or stage cancer, includes:
    a. Incisional biopsy: removing a portion of tumor tissue for examination
    b. Excisional biopsy: removing an entire tumor for examination
    c. Needle biopsy: using a needle to aspirate tissue or fluid for examination
    d. Endoscopic procedure: using an endoscope to examine internal tissues; e.g., diagnostic laparoscopy to examine the abdominal cavity
    e. Diagnostic laparotomy: creating a surgical opening in the abdomen to examine the abdominal cavity
    f. Second-look procedure: confirming the presence or absence of a tumor after original treatment
6. *Curative surgery*, done to eradicate cancer, includes:
    a. Such procedures as electrosurgery, cryosurgery, chemosurgery, and carbon dioxide (CO_2) laser surgery for cancer in situ
    b. Local excision
    c. En bloc resection
7. *Palliative surgery*, done to alleviate symptoms, includes:
    a. Resection of solitary metastases; e.g., lung resection for a single metastasis to decrease tumor bulk and relieve pain or pressure on surrounding tissues
    b. Procedures to decompress vital structures; e.g., laminectomy to alleviate spinal cord compression
    c. Procedures to alleviate obstructions; e.g., creating an ostomy to alleviate small bowel obstruction
    d. Ablative surgery; e.g., oophorectomy to remove endogenous sources of estrogen and promote remission of metastatic breast cancer
    e. Neurosurgery; e.g., spinal cord block for pain management
8. *Prophylactic surgery*, done to remove organs or tissues that have a high risk of developing cancer, includes:
    a. Colectomy for ulcerative colitis to prevent colon cancer
    b. Hysterectomy for adenomatous hyperplasia to prevent endometrial cancer

9. *Reconstructive or rehabilitative surgery*, done to improve a patient's appearance or function, includes:
    a. Reconstruction of breast tissue after mastectomy
    b. Insertion of a penile implant to restore sexual function
    c. Reconstruction of resected limbs using bone grafts
10. *Mechanical device insertion*, done to facilitate treatment or patient comfort, includes:
    a. Insertion of venous access devices to provide access for drug delivery and eliminate the need for repeated venipunctures
    b. Insertion of arterial lines to provide access for drug delivery, facilitate collection of blood specimens, and eliminate the need for multiple punctures
    c. Insertion of intraperitoneal access devices to enable drug delivery and eliminate the need for multiple punctures
    d. Implantation of a ventricular reservoir to provide direct access to the ventricular cerebrospinal fluid and facilitate drug delivery into the subarachnoid space
    e. Implantation of radioactive implants to deliver regulated doses of radiation to specific sites
11. Mechanism of action of surgery
    a. Removal of the tumor mass reduces or alleviates the tumor burden
    b. Host defenses or adjuvant treatment can then eliminate residual disease
12. Possible adverse effects of cancer surgery
    a. Adverse effects depend on the type, extent, and duration of surgery and on the patient's health status
    b. Adverse effects may be *local*, such as delayed wound healing or cosmetic defects, or *systemic*, such as fluid and electrolyte imbalance, hemorrhage, or malnutrition
13. *General* nursing interventions for patients undergoing surgery
    a. Explain the rationale, plan, and goal of surgery to the patient
    b. Explain all preoperative procedures, such as bowel preparation and laboratory studies
    c. Discuss what the patient can expect after surgery; e.g., describe the recovery room, explain what I.V. lines and catheters may be in place, describe the appearance of the surgical incision, and explain the pain the patient may experience
    d. Discuss the activities that the patient will be expected to perform after surgery to prevent postoperative complications; e.g., turning, coughing, deep breathing, and early ambulation
    e. Describe the care that the patient can expect from health care personnel following surgery; e.g., assistance with activities of daily living and administration of pain medications
    f. Verify completion of required preoperative tests, such as blood tests and X-rays
    g. Review the patient's chart to make sure all test results are recorded

    h. Assist the patient with preoperative preparations, such as enema, douche, and skin scrub

    i. After surgery, monitor vital signs for changes or abnormalities

    j. Assess function of I.V. lines, drains, and catheters for potential problems

    k. Check incisional dressings for drainage

    l. Assess for signs and symptoms of bleeding; e.g., monitor pulse rate and output from drainage devices

    m. Assess for signs and symptoms of infection

    n. Provide pain medications for patient comfort as ordered and as needed

    o. Administer I.V. fluids, as ordered, to maintain homeostasis

    p. Assess fluid and electrolyte balance by monitoring intake and output and evaluating laboratory results

    q. Provide aggressive pulmonary care—e.g., turning, coughing, and deep breathing—to prevent pulmonary complications

    r. Maintain nutritional intake; advance diet, as ordered

    s. Administer other medications, such as antibiotics, as ordered

14. *Specific* nursing interventions for patients undergoing cancer surgery (addresses key areas of nutrition, hemostasis, emotional support, effects of previous treatment, and rehabilitation)

    a. Evaluate the actual and potential impact of cancer and cancer surgery on the physical, psychosocial, and cognitive status of the patient and family

    b. Evaluate any adverse effects of previous treatment and their implications for proposed surgery; e.g., fibrosis secondary to radiation therapy may lead to poor wound healing

    c. Discuss with the patient the possible impact of previous treatments on current surgery

    d. Take steps to prevent complications when possible; e.g., be sure that neutropenia caused by chemotherapy is corrected before surgery

    e. Assess nutritional status; the patient may be nutritionally debilitated from cancer or previous treatment (see Section IV for specific information on nutrition and cancer)

    f. Monitor for signs and symptoms of nutritional deficiencies, which increase the risk of poor wound healing, pneumonia, and infection

    g. As ordered, administer enteral supplements and parenteral nutrition to reverse malnutrition

    h. Keep in mind that cancer patients may develop altered coagulation, possibly leading to such problems as disseminated intravascular coagulation or thromboembolism during or after surgery

    i. Assess hemodynamic status by monitoring vital signs and central venous pressure

    j. As ordered, help reduce the risk of thromboembolism by applying antiembolism stockings, administering prophylactic anticoagulants, and encouraging early ambulation

   k. Express realistic goals for surgery; e.g., tell a patient undergoing palliative surgery to expect some symptom relief, but not cure
   l. Encourage the patient to express his feelings about the cancer and the surgery
   m. Teach the patient about the cancer, its treatment, and possible adverse effects of treatment to help alleviate any anxiety caused by lack of knowledge
   n. Evaluate any disfigurement or debilitation caused by surgery and consider its impact on the patient. Keep in mind that some types of surgery—e.g., ostomy formation—alter body function and can cause significant changes in the patient's body image
   o. Help the patient regain a healthful self-image and return to a normal life-style by recommending reconstruction or rehabilitation resources, such as ostomy, laryngectomy, or breast cancer support groups, when appropriate
   p. As necessary, refer the patient to multidisciplinary health care team members, such as a chaplain or social worker

C. Radiation therapy
   1. General information
      a. Radiation therapy (RT) involves the use of high energy radiation to treat cancer
      b. RT may be used alone or in conjunction with other cancer treatment modalities
      c. RT is used primarily to treat localized cancers
      d. Radiation dosage in RT is measured in radiation absorbed dose (rad) or centigray (cGy); 1 rad equals 1 cGy
   2. Guiding principle for RT: The radiation dose administered should be large enough to eradicate the tumor but small enough to minimize the adverse effects to surrounding normal tissue; known as the *therapeutic ratio*
   3. Goals of RT
      a. Patient cure
      b. Disease control
      c. Symptom palliation
      d. Prophylactic treatment; e.g., irradiating the brain to prevent metastasis of small cell lung cancer
      e. Prophylactic palliation of impending symptoms; e.g., irradiating a mediastinal mass to prevent obstruction
   4. Factors affecting patient response to RT
      a. Degree of tissue oxygenation: Well oxygenated tissues are more radiosensitive than poorly oxygenated tissues
      b. Type of linear energy transfer (LET): Low LET radiation (e.g., X-rays and gamma rays) results in limited tumor penetration and limited cell damage; high LET radiation (e.g., alpha particles and neutrons) results in deeper penetration, more "direct" hits, and greater cellular damage

    c. Type of radiation therapy: Different types of RT— external beam therapy, brachytherapy, interstitial implants, and systemic irradiation—require different doses to achieve similar biologic effects

    d. Dose rate: Low dose rates are considered less effective than high dose rates for cell kill because low dose rates permit cellular repair before lethal doses are achieved

    e. Sensitivity of cells to RT: Proliferating cells are more radiosensitive than nonproliferating cells (e.g., cells in the GI tract are more radiosensitive than muscle cells), and poorly differentiated cells are more radiosensitive than well differentiated cells (e.g., stem cells of red blood cells are more radiosensitive than mature erythrocytes)

    f. Fractionation: The manner in which the total radiation dose is divided affects the radiosensitivity of some tumor cells

    g. Tissue response: "Direct" hits on the tumor cause cell death, and irradiation of supporting tissues can indirectly cause tumor cell death by destroying supportive vasculature

    h. Host factors: previous treatments, physical stature, and extent of disease

5. Types of radiation used in RT
    a. Electromagnetic radiation: radiation in wave form, such as X-rays, electrons, and gamma rays
    b. Particulate radiation: radiation in heavy particle form
    c. Alpha particulate radiation: positively charged particles; poor tissue penetration
    d. Beta particulate radiation: high-speed electrons; better tissue penetration than alpha particulate radiation
    e. Pion (pimeson) particulate radiation: unstable nuclear particles; good tissue penetration
    f. Neutron particulate radiation: uncharged particles; good tissue penetration

6. Types of RT
    a. External beam therapy (teletherapy): radiation source is outside the body
    b. Brachytherapy: radiation source is placed directly on the body surface or positioned near the body area being treated
    c. Interstitial RT: radiation source is implanted into involved tissues
    d. Systemic RT: radiation source is absorbed into the circulation and travels throughout the body

7. Mechanisms of action of RT
    a. RT causes cellular damage
    b. "Direct" hits damage molecules within the cell, such as DNA or RNA molecules; unrepaired molecular damage causes impaired cell function or cell death
    c. "Indirect" hits ionize the medium (primarily water) surrounding cell macromolecules, possibly causing molecular damage or a change in cell membrane permeability

    d. Radiation may delay or completely inhibit mitosis. Delayed onset of mitosis permits cellular repair; complete inhibition results in cell death resulting from the cell's inability to propagate

8. Possible adverse effects of RT
    a. Early effects—such as anorexia, nausea, diarrhea, and mucositis—occur during treatment and within the first 6 months after treatment, and usually result from disrupted mitotic activity
    b. Late effects—such as pulmonary fibrosis, radiation nephritis, atrophic gastritis, and intestinal obstruction—occur more than 6 months after treatment and result from cells attempting to repair damage caused by radiation
    c. Adverse effects are related to radiation dose delivered within a specific time period, method of RT delivery, and the patient's overall health status
    d. Adverse effects are limited to the treatment site; e.g., alopecia resulting from RT to the scalp, nausea and vomiting from RT to the abdomen, and diarrhea and cystitis from RT to the pelvis

9. Safety guidelines for brachytherapy and interstitial and systemic RT
    a. Radiation safety is based on the principle of minimizing radiation exposure by maintaining a safe distance and the shielding between persons and radioactive sources
    b. Specific safety procedures depend on the type of radiation, half-life of the radioisotope, dose, and method of administration

10. Safety measures to protect nurses and others during interstitial RT
    a. Keep in mind that a patient with an implanted radioisotope is radioactive
    b. Make sure the patient is in a private room
    c. Organize nursing activities to minimize the time spent in the patient's room
    d. Use the intercom to communicate with the patient whenever possible
    e. When in the patient's room, maintain the maximum possible distance from the patient
    f. Mark the patient's room and chart with radiation safety labels
    g. Limit the time that any visitors spend with the patient
    h. Do not permit children or pregnant women into the patient's room
    i. Encourage the patient to perform as many self-care activities as possible
    j. Check linens, bedpans, and other items for signs of dislodged implant. If you find any, contact the hospital's radiation safety or RT department
    k. Never touch a dislodged implant; instead, use tongs to place it in a protective safety container, which should be in the patient's room

11. Safety measures to protect nurses and others in systemically administered RT
    a. Because a systemically administered radioisotope may cause radioactive body secretions, wear gloves when handling the patient's body secretions or items that come in contact with body secretions
    b. Use disposable food trays and utensils

      c. Keep linens and trash in the patient's room until they have been checked for radioactivity by radiation therapy personnel

      d. See Section II.C.10 above for additional safety measures

  12. General nursing interventions for patients receiving RT

      a. Evaluate the actual and potential impact of cancer and RT on the physical, psychosocial, and cognitive status of the patient and family

      b. Teach the patient and family the rationale, goals, plan, and possible adverse effects of treatment

      c. Teach the patient and family how to manage adverse effects of treatment

      d. Explain possible aspects of the treatment plan, such as simulation, daily treatment, need to isolate patients with implants, and outpatient-inpatient settings

      e. Help the patient and family arrange transportation to and from treatment sessions, if necessary

      f. Provide psychosocial support as necessary

      g. Assess hydration and nutrition and help the patient maintain fluid and electrolyte balance

      h. Assess the patient's financial situation and refer to appropriate resources for assistance

      i. As necessary, refer the patient to appropriate multidisciplinary health care team members, such as a chaplain or nutritionist

      j. Provide for adequate safety measures (see Sections II.C.9, II.C.10, and II.C.11)

D. Chemotherapy

  1. General information

      a. Cancer chemotherapy is a systemic treatment modality involving the administration of antineoplastic agents

      b. Chemotherapy may be used alone or in conjunction with other cancer treatment modalities

      c. Chemotherapy functions at the cellular level and affects both normal cells and cancer cells

      d. Decisions on chemotherapy are based on the biology of the cancer (its cell type, growth rate, and extent of growth); treatment goals; the patient's clinical condition; the patient's drug allergies; pharmacologic action and effectiveness of available drugs; and the patient's desired quality of life

  2. Guiding principle for chemotherapy: Cancer chemotherapy aims to administer an antineoplastic agent dose large enough to eradicate cancer cells but small enough to limit adverse effects to safe and tolerable levels; known as the *therapeutic ratio*

  3. Goals of chemotherapy

      a. Patient cure

      b. Disease control

      c. Symptom palliation

4. Routes of administration
   a. Oral
   b. Intramuscular and subcutaneous injection
   c. I.V. infusion through veins and implanted venous access devices
   d. Intra-arterial infusion
   e. Intracavitary infusion, such as into the bladder, peritoneum, pleura, or pericardium
   f. Intrathecal injection (into the subarachnoid space of the spinal cord)
   g. Instillation through a ventricular reservoir
   h. Topical application
5. Equipment used to administer chemotherapy
   a. External venous access devices, such as the Hickman catheter
   b. Implanted venous access devices, such as the Port-A-Cath and the Infuse-A-Port
   c. Portable external infusion pumps, such as CorMed and Pharmacia CADD pumps
   d. Nonportable external infusion pumps, such as the I-med pump
   e. Implanted infusion pumps, such as the Infusaid pump
   f. Cerebrospinal fluid reservoirs, such as the Ommaya reservoir
   g. External peritoneal access devices, such as the external Tenckhoff catheter
   h. Implanted peritoneal access devices, such as the intraperitoneal port
6. Mechanisms of action of chemotherapy
   a. Most antineoplastic agents disrupt DNA synthesis
   b. Chemotherapy has its greatest effects on rapidly dividing cells, such as cells of the mucous membranes and bone marrow. It affects both normal cells and cancer cells, but while normal cells can repair themselves, cancer cells are less able to do so
7. Possible adverse effects of chemotherapy
   a. Adverse effects result from the action of antineoplastic agents on all rapidly dividing cells
   b. Specific adverse effects depend on the type of agent administered
8. Safety guidelines for preparing and administering chemotherapy (recommendations developed in 1984 by the National Study Commission on Cytotoxic Exposure to prevent or minimize drug absorption from direct skin contact and inhalation)
   a. Prepare injectable antineoplastic agents under a class II vertical laminar flow biologic safety cabinet with a filtered exhaust to the outdoors
   b. Cover work surfaces with plastic-backed absorbent paper to minimize dispersion of any spills
   c. When preparing drugs, wear a closed-front surgical gown with knit or elastic cuffs and surgical latex gloves; do not use polyvinyl-chloride gloves because many drugs can permeate them
   d. Minimize drug aerosolization during preparation by venting vials or by placing alcohol-soaked cotton or gauze pads at the necks of ampules

    e. After preparing antineoplastic agents, clean all work surfaces, remove gown and gloves, and dispose of all materials in accordance with regulations and procedures governing toxic and chemical waste disposal

    f. When administering antineoplastic agents, wear a surgical gown with knit or elastic cuffs and surgical latex gloves

    g. To minimize aerosolization during administration, place alcohol-soaked gauze pads over tips of needles or I.V. tubing when removing air

    h. Dispose of all equipment used to administer antineoplastic agents in accordance with regulations and procedures governing toxic and chemical waste disposal

    i. If antineoplastic agents come in contact with skin, immediately wash the affected area with soap and water

    j. Wear protective clothing and two pairs of surgical latex gloves when cleaning any spills

    k. Wear surgical latex gloves when handling the excreta of patients who have received antineoplastic agents

    l. Wash your hands thoroughly after preparing or administering any antineoplastic agent and handling any patient excreta

9. Extravasation of injected antineoplastic agents

    a. Antineoplastic agents leaking from blood vessels may cause local tissue damage, ranging from mild irritation, inflammation, and burning to severe ulceration and necrosis

    b. Tissue damage depends on the particular agent, the amount of extravasation, and the duration of exposure

    c. Possible causes of extravasation include small or fragile blood vessels, elevated venous pressure due to hypertension, edema, superior vena cava syndrome, and poor venipuncture technique

    d. Previously irradiated tissue may be prone to extravasation

    e. Cases of severe extravasation may require surgical consultation for tissue debridement and repair

10. Guidelines to prevent or minimize extravasation

    a. Avoid injection into vessels near nerves and tendons

    b. Avoid using multiple puncture sites in the same vessel

    c. If multiple punctures in one vessel are necessary, start at a distal point on the extremity and make subsequent punctures at progressively proximal points

11. General nursing interventions for patients receiving chemotherapy

    a. Evaluate the actual and potential impact of cancer and chemotherapy on the physical, psychosocial, and cognitive status of the patient and family

    b. Monitor the patient's physical condition for factors that may affect his ability to tolerate chemotherapy, such as changes in bone marrow, hepatic, cardiac, or renal function

c. Review records of previous treatments to guard against possible synergistic or additive adverse effects, such as from cumulative doses or recall phenomenon

d. Discuss with the patient and family the rationale, goals, plan, logistics, and possible adverse effects of treatment

e. Teach the patient and family how to manage adverse effects of treatment

f. Inform the patient and family about symptoms, such as fever and pain, that should be reported to the health care team

g. Help the patient and family arrange transportation for treatment sessions

h. Provide psychosocial support as necessary

i. Help the patient maintain adequate hydration and nutrition

j. As necessary, refer the patient to appropriate multidisciplinary health care team members, such as a chaplain or social worker

Points to Remember

Cancer treatment modalities include surgery, radiation therapy (RT), and chemotherapy. These modalities may be used alone or in combination with one another.

Nursing interventions for patients undergoing cancer surgery are similar to those for patients undergoing surgery for benign conditions, with a particular emphasis on nutrition, hemostasis, emotional support, and rehabilitation.

RT can produce both early and late adverse effects.

RT safety measures for health care personnel depend on the type of radiation used.

The therapeutic ratio is the guiding treatment principle in RT and chemotherapy.

Health care personnel follow specific safety procedures for preparing and administering antineoplastic agents and handling chemotherapy waste products.

Glossary

Cytotoxic—destructive to cells

En bloc resection—surgical removal of a tumor or organ along with a wide margin of surrounding tissue, done to ensure removal of all tumor cells and prevent tumor dissemination

Extravasation—leakage of drug from a blood vessel

Fractionation—administering a radiation dose in smaller amounts over a period of time rather than in a single large dose

Linear energy transfer (LET)—rate of energy loss by radiation as it travels through matter

"No touch" technique—surgical technique involving minimal tumor manipulation to decrease the risk of tumor dissemination

Radiation dose—amount of radiation administered during a specific treatment period

Simulation—initial step in treatment planning for external beam RT, involving identification of tumor volume area through diagnostic testing and marking of the patient's skin to outline tumor volume and identify area to be irradiated

Antineoplastic Agents

Learning Objectives

After studying this section, the reader should be able to:

- Explain the rationale for using antineoplastic agents in cancer treatment.

- List the major adverse reactions associated with each antineoplastic agent.

- Identify important nursing interventions for a patient receiving an antineoplastic agent.

- Discuss important teaching points for a patient receiving an antineoplastic agent.

III. Antineoplastic Agents

A. Introduction

1. Mechanism of action
   a. Antineoplastic agents kill or inhibit reproduction of cancer cells
   b. Their effects may not be limited to cancer cells
   c. *Cell cycle-specific* agents affect cells only in a specific phase of the reproductive cycle; *cell cycle-nonspecific* agents affect cells in all phases of the reproductive cycle
2. Indications
   a. Antineoplastic agents are used to treat many solid tumors, lymphomas, and leukemias
   b. Agents usually are administered in combination to increase response and minimize toxicity
   c. They may be used in conjunction with other treatment modalities, such as surgery or radiation therapy (RT)
3. Contraindications and precautions
   a. Use is contraindicated in patients with previous bone marrow suppression and in pregnant or lactating patients
   b. Antineoplastic agents should be administered cautiously in patients with decreased bone marrow reserve or infections, patients receiving RT, and patients who may become pregnant during the course of therapy
4. Possible adverse reactions result from the drugs' action on all rapidly dividing cells, such as those of the bone marrow, mucous membranes, GI tract, and hair follicles
5. Nursing interventions
   a. Assessment: monitor complete blood count, cell differential, and platelet count; assess for nausea and vomiting; assess for phlebitis and extravasation at injection sites
   b. Implementation: prepare parenteral antineoplastic agents in a class II laminar flow biologic safety cabinet; wear gloves, gown, and mask while handling agents; discard administration equipment according to protocol in designated containers; avoid giving intramuscular injections or taking temperature rectally; administer antineoplastics in high-dose, intermittent courses to maximize effects while permitting recovery of normal cells; maintain patient's fluid intake at a minimum of 2,000 ml/day; adminster antiemetics, as needed; follow treatment protocol for extravasation
   c. Evaluation: base evaluation of patient response on degree of reduction in cancer size and spread and occurrence of toxic adverse reactions
6. Patient teaching
   a. Tell the patient to notify the physician immediately if fever, sore throat, signs of infection, or unusual bleeding occur
   b. Instruct the patient to avoid crowds and persons known to have infections
   c. Instruct the patient to use a soft toothbrush and an electric razor to minimize the risk of gum and skin irritation and bleeding
   d. Warn the patient to avoid products containing alcohol and aspirin

ANTINEOPLASTIC AGENTS AND THE CELL CYCLE

The cell cycle is divided into five distinct phases of replication:
- Phase G_0: the resting phase
- Phase G_1: RNA and protein synthesis
- Phase S: DNA synthesis
- Phase G_2: RNA and protein synthesis
- Phase M: mitosis—cell division

    Antineoplastic agents stop cancer cell production by interrupting the cell cycle. *Cell cycle-specific agents,* such as methotrexate, act only at particular cell cycle phases. *Cell cycle-nonspecific agents,* such as busulfan, can act at several or all cell cycle phases. This diagram of the cell cycle lists common antineoplastic agents under the phase or phases in which they exert their actions.

S
methotrexate
fluorouracil
mercaptopurine
cytarabine

G_2
bleomycin
sulfate

M
etoposide (VP-16)
vinblastine sulfate
vincristine sulfate
busulfan
vindesine sulfate

G_1
asparaginase

G_0
lomustine
busulfan
carmustine

    e. Tell the patient to consult the physician before receiving any vaccinations or taking any new medications

    f. For a patient receiving an agent known to cause alopecia, discuss the possibility of hair loss and methods of coping with this problem

    g. As appropriate, discuss with the patient and patient's partner the need for contraception because of the teratogenic effects of many agents

    h. Instruct a patient at risk for stomatitis to inspect the oral mucosa regularly for erythema and ulceration, use a sponge toothbrush, and rinse his mouth after meals and at bedtime; if stomatitis occurs, instruct the patient to rinse his mouth with a sodium chloride solution or stomatitis "cocktail" preparation every 2 hours during the day and every 6 hours at night

B. Alkylating agents

  1. Drug examples

    a. Busulfan (Myleran)

    b. Chlorambucil (Leukeran)

    c. Cisplatin (Platinol)

    d. Cyclophosphamide (Cytoxan, Neosar)

    e. Mechlorethamine (Mustargen)

  2. Mechanism of action: These *cell cycle-nonspecific* agents affect DNA synthesis by cross-linking DNA to inhibit cell reproduction

  3. Possible adverse reactions

    a. Alopecia (cyclophosphamide)

    b. Gonadal suppression (chlorambucil, cyclophosphamide, mechlorethamine)

    c. Hyperuricemia (busulfan, chlorambucil, mechlorethamine)

    d. Ototoxicity, tinnitus, hypomagnesemia, hypokalemia, hypocalcemia, nephrotoxicity (cisplatin)

    e. Hemorrhagic cystitis, hematuria (cyclophosphamide)

  4. Interactions

    a. Additive ototoxicity and nephrotoxicity occur with concomitant use of other ototoxic and nephrotoxic agents

    b. Phenobarbital may enhance the effects of cyclophosphamide

  5. Nursing interventions

    a. Monitor a patient receiving cisplatin for dizziness, tinnitus, hearing loss, loss of coordination, and numbness or tingling in arms and legs; these effects may be irreversible

    b. If extravasation occurs during mechlorethamine adminstration, immediately administer an injection of 1/16 molar sodium thiosulfate into the extravasation site to help prevent tissue necrosis

  6. Patient teaching

    a. Explain that the patient may be susceptible to easy bruising, infection, and fatigue because of these agents' effects on bone marrow function

    b. Instruct a patient receiving cisplatin to report any hearing problems

C. Antineoplastic antibiotics
1. Drug examples
   a. Bleomycin (Blenoxane)
   b. Dactinomycin (Actinomycin-D, Cosmegen)
   c. Daunorubicin (Cerubidine)
   d. Doxorubicin (Adriamycin)
2. Mechanism of action: These *cell cycle-nonspecific* agents interfere with DNA and RNA synthesis
3. Possible adverse reactions
   a. Alopecia, stomatitis, phlebitis at I.V. infusion site, gonadal suppression, hyperuricemia (all antitumor antibiotics)
   b. Congestive heart failure, dysrhythmias (daunorubicin)
   c. Cardiomyopathy, ECG changes (doxorubicin)
4. Interactions
   a. Adminstering daunorubicin concomitantly with other hepatotoxic drugs increases the risk of hepatotoxicity
   b. Mixing heparin sodium or dexamethasone phosphate with daunorubicin or doxorubicin may cause precipitate formation
5. Nursing interventions
   a. Monitor vital signs frequently during administration
   b. Assess a patient receiving daunorubicin for signs of congestive heart failure, such as dyspnea, crackles, peripheral edema, and weight gain
   c. Assess a patient receiving doxorubicin for signs of myocardial toxicity, such as dyspnea, dysrhythmias, hypotension, and weight gain
6. Patient teaching
   a. Inform the patient that dactinomycin may cause alopecia but that this effect usually is reversible after cessation of therapy
   b. Warn the patient that urine may appear red-tinged for a day or two following therapy with daunorubicin or doxorubicin

D. Antimetabolites
1. Drug examples
   a. Cytarabine (ARA-C, cytosine arabinoside, Cytosar-U)
   b. Fluorouracil (5-FU, Adrucil, Efudex, Fluoroplex)
   c. Mercaptopurine (6-MP, Purinethol)
   d. Methotrexate (Folex, Mexate)
2. Mechanism of action: These *cell cycle-specific* agents replace the normal protein required for DNA synthesis
3. Possible adverse reactions
   a. Alopecia (cytarabine, fluorouracil, methotrexate)
   b. Stomatitis (cytarabine, fluorouracil, methotrexate)
   c. Hyperuricemia (cytarabine, mercaptopurine, methotrexate)
   d. Diarrhea (fluorouracil)
   e. Hepatotoxicity (cytarabine, mercaptopurine, methotrexate)
   f. Photosensitivity (fluorouracil, methotrexate)

4. Interactions
   a. Administering mercaptopurine and methotrexate concomitantly with other hepatotoxic agents results in additive hepatotoxicity
   b. Allopurinol inhibits metabolism of mercaptopurine and increases the risk of toxicity
   c. Salicylates, oral hypoglycemic agents, phenytoin, phenylbutazone, tetracyclines, probenecid, and chloramphenicol increase the risk of methotrexate toxicity
5. Nursing interventions
   a. Assess a patient receiving fluorouracil for symptoms of cerebellar dysfunction such as dizziness, weakness, and ataxia, and for stomatitis and diarrhea. Presence of stomatitis and diarrhea may necessitate discontinuation of therapy or change in dosage
   b. Ensure that a patient receiving high doses of methotrexate also receives folinic acid or citrovorum factor (Leucovorin rescue) to prevent potentially fatal toxicity
6. Patient teaching: Instruct a patient receiving fluorouracil or methotrexate to use a sunscreen and wear protective clothing when exposed to sunlight, in order to prevent photosensitivity reactions

E. **Hormonal antineoplastic agents**
   1. Drug examples
      a. Diethylstilbestrol (DES)
      b. Megestrol (Megace, Pallace)
      c. Prednisone (Deltasone)
      d. Tamoxifen (Nolvadex)
      e. Testosterone (Andro, Depo-Testosterone, Testex)
   2. Mechanism of action
      a. Interferes with or blocks the binding of normal hormones to receptor proteins; manipulates hormone levels and alters the hormonal environment of the tumor cell, possibly resulting in suppression of tumor growth
      b. May cause immunosuppression
   3. Possible adverse reactions
      a. Edema, hypercalcemia (diethylstilbestrol, tamoxifen, testosterone)
      b. Impotence, gynecomastia in men (diethylstilbestrol)
   4. Interactions
      a. Diethylstilbestrol and testosterone may alter the effects of oral anticoagulants, oral hypoglycemic agents, and insulin
      b. Tamoxifen reduces the effectiveness of estrogen
   5. Nursing interventions
      a. Monitor serum calcium levels of a patient receiving tamoxifen or testosterone, which may cause hypercalcemia in patients with bone metastasis
      b. Observe a female patient receiving testosterone for signs of virilization

  c. Observe a male patient receiving megesterol or diethylstilbestrol for signs of gynecomastia

  d. Monitor a patient receiving prednisone for signs of infection or delayed wound healing

  e. Discontinue prednisone therapy gradually, to prevent withdrawal symptoms

 6. Patient teaching

  a. Warn a patient receiving tamoxifen that he may experience severe bone pain; explain that this indicates that the drug is effective, and reassure him that the pain will subside in time and that analgesics can help control pain

  b. Warn against discontinuing prednisone abruptly or without physician's consent

F. Vinca alkaloids

 1. Drug examples

  a. Vinblastine (Velban)

  b. Vincristine (Oncovin)

  c. Vindesine (Eldisine); available in Canada only

 2. Mechanism of action: These *cell cycle-specific* agents prevent mitosis

 3. Possible adverse reactions (all agents)

  a. Peripheral neuropathy, hyperuricemia

  b. Stomatitis, anorexia, constipation, phlebitis at I.V. site

  c. Alopecia

 4. Interactions

  a. Combining vincristine with other chemotherapeutic agents may increase the cytotoxic effects of these agents

  b. Combining vinca alkaloids with other neurotoxic drugs creates an additive effect that increases neurotoxicity

 5. Nursing interventions

  a. Assess for signs and symptoms of neurotoxicity, such as neuromuscular abnormalities and constipation

  b. Keep in mind that a patient with a history of liver disease may require dosage adjustments

  c. Remember that vincristine may exacerbate pre-existing neurologic problems

  d. If extravasation occurs during vinca alkaloid administration, immediately inject hyaluronidase into the extravasation site; do not inject steroids or apply cold compresses (Keep in mind that this intervention is controversial)

 6. Patient teaching

  a. Instruct the patient to watch for and report any signs and symptoms of neurotoxicity or drug extravasation

  b. Encourage the patient receiving vinca alkaloids to drink plenty of fluids to increase uric acid excretion and prevent hyperuricemia

Points to Remember

Antineoplastic agents kill tumor cells or inhibit their reproduction.

Antineoplastic agents are either cell cycle-specific or cell cycle-nonspecific.

Adverse reactions to antineoplastic agents, such as bone marrow suppression, anorexia, nausea, vomiting, alopecia, stomatitis, and gonadal suppression, result when these agents damage rapidly dividing normal cells.

Patient teaching should address contraception during treatment, physiologic and psychologic effects of treatment, problems requiring physician notification, and prevention of adverse reactions.

Glossary

Alopecia—loss of hair

Bone marrow suppression—reduced blood cell production caused by hematologic toxicity; can result in thrombocytopenia, leukopenia, or anemia

Cross-linking—deactivating DNA by creating bonds that cause abnormal base pairing

Gonadal suppression—reduction in the number or function of reproductive cells

Stomatitis—inflammation, with the potential for ulceration, of the oral mucosa

Nutrition and Cancer

Learning Objectives

After studying this section, the reader should be able to:

● Identify possible cancer-related causes of decreased nutrient intake.

● Describe factors that influence the choice of nutritional support therapy.

● Discuss changes in nutrient metabolism that may occur in cancer patients.

● Discuss possible effects of cancer treatment on nutritional status.

● Describe the components of a nutritional assessment.

● Discuss nursing interventions to provide nutritional support.

IV. Nutrition and Cancer

A. Introduction

1. Most cancer patients experience nutritional imbalance
2. Comparing a patient's increased nutritional requirements to actual nutritional intake determines the nature of this imbalance
3. A cancer patient may require increased intake of:
   a. Carbohydrates, to meet increased metabolic demands
   b. Calories, for tissue repair
   c. Protein, for tissue repair and wound healing
4. A cancer patient often receives some form of nutritional support therapy to meet these increased requirements
5. Choice of a specific nutritional support therapy depends on goals of therapy, such as promoting weight gain, maintaining current weight, or prolonging life
6. A patient's nutrient and caloric requirements are identified to help meet the goals of therapy
7. Other factors affecting the choice of nutritional support therapy include:
   a. The patient's ability to chew and swallow
   b. Status of the patient's GI tract
   c. Severity of the nutritional problem
   d. Complications resulting from other cancer treatment modalities
   e. Cost of therapy and patient's financial resources
   f. Duration of therapy
   g. Patient consent and cooperation
   h. Availability of support persons, such as family or friends

B. Possible cancer-related causes of nutritional imbalance

1. General information
   a. Cancer cells compete with host for available nutrients
   b. Cancer, the treatment modality, and the patient's physiologic and psychological response to cancer or its treatment may increase nutritional demands
   c. Basal metabolic rate increases
   d. Protein and fat reserves become depleted
   e. Dietary intake may be insufficient to meet increased nutritional demands
2. Effects of cancer on nutritional status
   a. A tumor may cause mechanical interference with the ability to eat or the body's ability to utilize nutrients
   b. A tumor's metabolic demand may exceed the patient's nutrient intake; if prolonged, this may result in *cachexia*
   c. Cancer patients often experience *glycolysis* and increased *gluconeogenesis*; increased gluconeogenesis contributes to protein-calorie malnutrition

    d. Protein synthesis decreases because the body cannot use insulin appropriately; instead, the body uses skeletal muscle as a protein source for energy production, which leads to muscle wasting, protein loss, and negative nitrogen balance

    e. Lipolysis provides energy when caloric intake drops and insulin use changes; this process depletes the body's fat reserves

3. Effects of cancer surgery on nutritional status

    a. Fluid loss during surgery causes fluid and electrolyte imbalance

    b. Head or neck surgery to remove vital structures, postoperative edema, or the need to avoid postoperative suture line tension may interfere with the patient's ability to eat

    c. Bowel resection surgery prohibits oral intake while suture lines heal

    d. Manipulation of the GI tract during surgery causes postoperative gastric stasis and ileus

    e. Resection of organs that secrete digestive enzymes or a bowel section that normally absorbs nutrients may inhibit absorption of lipids, protein, and vitamins

    f. Partial bowel resection or gastric surgery may cause dumping syndrome

    g. Pancreas resection may cause diabetes mellitus

4. Effects of radiation therapy (RT) on nutritional status depend on the type and site of irradiation

    a. Fatigue and circulating tumor wastes may cause anorexia

    b. GI tract irritation may cause nausea and vomiting

    c. Decreased saliva production and alterations in saliva components that protect teeth may cause dental caries

    d. Destruction of salivary glands causes dry mouth syndrome

    e. Dry mouth, edema, and mucositis may cause dysphagia

    f. Irritation or destruction of taste buds may alter the sense of taste

    g. Irritation or destruction of oral mucosa may cause gingivitis

    h. Edema and cell destruction in the esophagus may cause esophagitis

    i. Irritation or cell destruction in the GI mucosa may cause mucositis, enteritis, or diarrhea

    j. Destruction of normal and tumor tissue and improper wound healing may cause fistula formation

5. Effects of chemotherapy on nutritional status

    a. Combination chemotherapy increases the risk of nutritional imbalance

    b. Depression, fatigue, or circulating tumor wastes may cause anorexia

    c. GI tract irritation or drug stimulation of the true vomiting center and chemoreceptor trigger zone may cause nausea and vomiting

    d. Irritation or destruction of oral mucosa may cause stomatitis

    e. Irritation or destruction of taste buds may alter the sense of taste

    f. Edema, irritation, or cell destruction in the esophagus may cause esophagitis

    g. Edema, irritation, or cell destruction in the GI tract may cause enteritis, mucositis, or diarrhea

C. Nutritional assessment
1. Measure height and weight
   a. Compare height and weight to ideal height and ideal body weight (IBW) on standard charts
   b. Note any significant weight loss (a loss exceeding 10% of preillness weight)
   c. Question patient about any changes in fit of clothing
2. Obtain a dietary history that includes:
   a. Types of food usually eaten and meal frequency
   b. Food preferences
   c. Dental problems
   d. Current medications
   e. Recent treatments
   f. Adverse effects of treatment and any related eating difficulties
   g. Measures taken to control adverse effects
3. Obtain a 24-hour dietary recall
4. Measure skinfold thickness and mid-arm muscle circumference
5. Evaluate results of laboratory tests that reflect nutritional status
   a. Serum albumin: <3.2 g/dl may indicate low protein stores, dehydration, or liver dysfunction
   b. Serum transferrin: >250 mg/dl may indicate iron deficiency; <200 mg/dl may indicate malnutrition
   c. Total lymphocyte count: <1,500 cells/mm^3 may indicate bone marrow suppression or malnutrition
   d. Urinary creatinine excretion: <18 to 23 mg/kg of IBW may indicate a low or insufficient amount of lean body mass
   e. Urinary urea nitrogen excretion: decreased excretion rate (normal rate is 9 to 20 mg/dl) may indicate protein depletion
   f. Skin tests of immune system function: negative reactions may indicate nutritional depletion

D. Nutritional support therapy: Oral
1. General information
   a. Used for patients with no swallowing impairment
   b. Accommodates various food forms; e.g., liquids and pureed foods for patients having difficulty chewing, and bland foods for patients with stomatitis
   c. Least expensive form of nutritional support therapy
2. Nursing interventions
   a. Emphasize the need for a high-protein, high-calorie diet
   b. Suggest ways to improve nutrition without adding bulk, such as mixing powdered milk in whole milk
   c. Suggest using natural or commercial nutritional supplements
   d. Perform a complete calorie count

E. **Nutritional support therapy: Enteral tube feedings**
   1. General information
      a. Used for patients with intact GI tract function
      b. Less expensive than peripheral parenteral nutrition
      c. May be administered through a nasogastric tube, gastrostomy tube, or jejunostomy tube
   2. Nursing interventions
      a. Check nasogastric tube placement before each feeding to prevent aspiration
      b. Elevate the head of bed before feeding to prevent aspiration
      c. Check tube patency by flushing with normal saline solution and aspirating, if ordered
      d. Feed the patient only during waking hours
      e. Make sure formula is at room temperature to prevent abdominal cramps
      f. Regulate feeding rate to prevent abdominal distention, nausea, vomiting, cramping, and diarrhea
      g. Provide skin care for nasogastric tube insertion site (nares) and gastrostomy and jejunostomy catheter sites to prevent skin damage and ulceration
      h. Involve the patient and family in the care program; e.g, by teaching them how to how to administer tube feedings and care for the catheter site

F. **Nutritional support therapy: Peripheral parenteral nutrition**
   1. General information
      a. Used to augment insufficient oral intake
      b. Used on a short-term basis in patients who are temporarily unable to tolerate oral or enteral tube feedings
      c. Contains 5% to 10% dextrose, amino acids, electrolytes, vitamins, and possibly 10% to 20% fat emulsion
      d. Does not meet a patient's total nutritional requirements
   2. Nursing interventions
      a. Monitor for signs and symptoms of thrombophlebitis and infiltration at the I.V. site
      b. Monitor complete blood count for signs of infection
      c. Assess for signs and symptoms of fluid overload
      d. Monitor for signs and symptoms of hyperglycemia—including elevated urine and blood glucose levels—which can result from a solution's high glucose concentration

G. **Nutritional support therapy: Total parenteral nutrition**
   1. General information
      a. Used for patients with GI tract dysfunction
      b. May be administered on a short- or long-term basis
      c. Contains 25% to 50% dextrose, amino acids, vitamins, trace elements, and possibly 10% to 20% fat emulsion
      d. May meet a patient's total nutritional requirements

2. Nursing interventions
    a. Before starting infusion, check X-rays to ensure proper catheter position, verify that each bottle contains the solution ordered, and evaluate each bottle for sterility
    b. Use sterile technique during infusion and dressing changes to prevent infection
    c. Regulate infusion rate with a volumetric pump to prevent fluid overload
    d. Increase infusion rate gradually to allow the patient time to adjust to changing blood glucose levels
    e. Monitor the catheter insertion site for signs and symptoms of local infection
    f. Interrupt total parenteral infusion (TPN) for blood work or other infusions only in emergencies; interruption increases the risk of infection
    g. Assess for signs and symptoms of systemic infection
    h. Assess for signs and symptoms of hyperglycemia or hypoglycemia; monitor serum glucose levels to detect hyperglycemia or hypoglycemia, and monitor urine glucose and acetone levels to detect hyperglycemia
    i. Measure and record weight daily; notify the physician of weight increase greater than 2 lb (1.0 kg) per day, which may indicate fluid retention or overload
    j. Change the catheter site dressing according to institutional protocol
    k. For patients receiving TPN in home care settings, teach the patient and family how to administer TPN, how to change dressings, and how to recognize adverse effects of TPN, such as the signs and symptoms of hyperglycemia and infection
    l. Teach the patient and family how to use home serum and urine glucose tests, such as a glucometer and urine dipsticks
    m. Explain that frequent laboratory blood tests are required to evaluate the need for changing solution contents
    n. Refer the patient to a visiting nurse association for home TPN care and monitoring

Points to Remember

Cancer and cancer therapy can adversely affect a patient's nutritional status.

Tumor cells compete with the host for available nutrients.

Decreased food intake and altered nutrient metabolism may cause nutritional deficiencies.

Tumors may cause mechanical interference with the patient's ability to consume or metabolize nutrients.

Enteral and parenteral supplements provide nutrients when the patient is unable to eat or cannot consume an adequate nutrient supply.

Glossary

Cachexia—state of general ill health and severe malnutrition marked by extreme weakness and emaciation

Gluconeogenesis—synthesis of glucose in the liver and renal cortex from noncarbohydrate sources, such as lactic acid and amino acids

Glycolysis—inefficient form of carbohydrate metabolism and energy production involving breakdown of glucose to yield lactic acid or pyruvic acid

Lipolysis—hydrolysis of triglycerides

Nursing Management of Common Cancer-Related Problems

Learning Objectives

After studying this section, the reader should be able to:

• Identify common problems experienced by cancer patients.

• Discuss possible causes of each problem.

• State several assessment findings for each problem.

• Identify possible nursing interventions to manage each problem.

V. Nursing Management of Common Cancer-Related Problems

A. **Introduction**
1. Cancer patients commonly experience problems resulting from the disease itself, its treatment, or the adverse effects of treatment
2. Nursing interventions for cancer patients are designed to prevent or minimize these problems

B. **Alopecia**
1. General information
   a. Alopecia refers to the temporary or permanent loss of body hair, especially on the scalp, face, axillae, and pubis
   b. It commonly occurs when radiation therapy (RT) or chemotherapy damages DNA in hair follicle stem cells
   c. The degree and duration of alopecia caused by chemotherapy depends on the drug and dosage
   d. The degree and duration of alopecia caused by RT depends on the radiation dose and treatment field; e.g., a radiation dose of 1500 to 3000 rads results in partial or complete temporary alopecia, with regrowth likely to involve changes in hair color and texture
2. Assessment findings
   a. Dry hair
   b. Brittle hair
   c. Hair on bed linens, clothes, furniture, or floor
   d. Thinning hair
   e. Patchy areas of hair on scalp
   f. Total hair loss
   g. Fine regrowth of hair between chemotherapy treatments
3. Nursing interventions
   a. Examine the patient's scalp
   b. Evaluate the extent and anticipated duration of hair loss, and inform the patient and family of your evaluation
   c. Explain that hair regrowth after temporary alopecia may differ from original color and texture
   d. Assess the anticipated impact of alopecia on the patient's life-style, especially in such areas as self-image, sexual identity and function, interpersonal relationships, and work and leisure activities
   e. Encourage the patient and family to express their anxieties and concerns related to alopecia
   f. Encourage the patient to purchase wigs, scarves, or hats before hair loss becomes extensive
   g. Prevent or minimize hair loss by inducing scalp hypothermia, using a device such as the Kay Kold Kap (when indicated)
   h. Prevent or minimize hair loss by using a tube or pneumatic scalp tourniquet (when indicated)

     i. Advise the patient to shampoo only every 3 to 5 days, using a mild, protein-based shampoo and cream rinse or conditioner, to help prevent hair dryness due to excessive washing

     j. Instruct the patient to pat, not rub, hair dry after shampooing to minimize manipulation of brittle hair

    k. Tell the patient to avoid excessive brushing to prevent tearing or unnecessary manipulation of hair

    l. Instruct the patient to discontinue use of electric hair dryers, rollers, irons or crimpers, hair clips, sprays, dyes, and permanents to prevent further hair damage

    m. Advise the patient to sleep on a satin pillow case to minimize hair tangles and friction

    n. As appropriate, encourage the patient to use makeup to minimize the noticeability of alopecia of the eyebrows and eyelashes

    o. Instruct the patient to cover his head to prevent sunburn in the summer and to minimize loss of body heat in the winter

C. Anemia
1. General information
   a. Anemia involves a deficiency in the amount of hemoglobin and number of erythrocytes in the blood
   b. Possible cancer- and cancer treatment-related causes include RT- or chemotherapy-induced myelosuppression, in which bone marrow stem cells fail to produce sufficient erythrocytes; hemolysis of erythrocytes by an antineoplastic agent; depletion of circulating erythrocytes from surgery; primary disease of the bone marrow, such as leukemia, that depresses erythrocyte formation or inhibits maturation; and secondary disease of the bone marrow, such as tumor infiltration replacing bone marrow
2. Assessment findings
   a. Pallor
   b. Weakness
   c. Fatigue
   d. Dyspnea
   e. Palpitations
   f. Listlessness
   g. Dizziness
   h. Headache
   i. Vertigo
   j. Depression
   k. Apathy
   l. Tachycardia
   m. Tachypnea
   n. Increased pulse pressure
   o. Decreased blood pressure
   p. Acute or chronic blood loss

q. Decreased hemoglobin and hematocrit
r. Decreased erythrocyte indices
s. Decreased erythrocyte and reticulocyte counts
t. Abnormal related laboratory test results, such as serum iron level
3. Nursing interventions
   a. Explain to the patient the causes and symptoms of anemia
   b. Teach and encourage safety measures, such as avoiding sudden changes of position and not driving if feeling faint
   c. Instruct the patient to notify the physician immediately if he develops overt gross bleeding, hematuria, hematemesis, or hematochezia
   d. Instruct the patient to maintain a diet high in protein, vitamins, and iron
   e. Encourage the patient to pace his activities to avoid fatigue, and to include adequate rest periods throughout the day
   f. Monitor laboratory test results, including erythrocyte and reticulocyte counts, hemoglobin and hematocrit, and serum iron level

D. Constipation
1. General information
   a. Constipation refers to difficult, irregular, or incomplete bowel movements involving discomfort or pain and hard feces
   b. It may result from physiologic conditions, such as GI tract tumors, adverse effects of treatment, narcotic use for pain relief, decreased mobility, and inability to consume adequate dietary roughage or psychological causes, such as anxiety and depression
2. Possible assessment findings
   a. Change in usual elimination pattern
   b. Decreased dietary fiber intake
   c. Decreased fluid intake
   d. Decrease in physical activity or mobility
   e. Abdominal distention
   f. Abdominal cramping
   g. Flatus
   h. Diminished bowel sounds
   i. Fecal impaction
3. Nursing interventions
   a. Explain the possible causes of constipation
   b. Teach measures to prevent constipation
   c. Encourage the patient to drink 3000 ml of fluid each day (unless contraindicated) to promote normal GI function
   d. Stress the importance of including high-fiber foods in the diet to promote GI motility
   e. Advise the patient to avoid foods that can cause constipation, such as dairy products and refined grain products
   f. Instruct the patient to increase physical activity, as tolerated, to promote GI motility

      g. Assess for and report abdominal distention or any change in bowel sounds
      h. Administer prophylactic stool softeners, as ordered
      i. Administer laxatives, suppositories, or enemas, as ordered
      j. Encourage the patient to defecate when the urge strikes; stress the importance of not delaying defecation
      k. Remove any fecal impaction as needed (unless contraindicated)

E. Diarrhea
1. General information
   a. Diarrhea refers to the abnormally frequent passage of soft or liquid stools
   b. Diarrhea results from disruption of normal water absorption in the large intestine. Possible cancer-and cancer treatment-related causes include GI tract tumors; destruction of the intestinal epithelial lining from surgery, RT, or chemotherapy; use of high-osmolarity nutritional supplements; and use of antibiotic drugs
2. Assessment findings
   a. Loose, frequent stools
   b. Emotional stress
   c. History of using a high-osmolarity nutritional supplement or an antibiotic drug
   d. Previous cancer treatment involving surgery, RT, or chemotherapy
   e. Abdominal distention
   f. Flatus
   g. Abdominal cramps
   h. Rectal irritation
   i. Hemorrhoid aggravation
   j. Dehydration
   k. Electrolyte imbalance
   l. Nutritional depletion
3. Nursing interventions
   a. Assess the patient's usual elimination patterns and evaluate for possible causes of diarrhea
   b. Assess for and report abdominal distention and any change in bowel sounds
   c. Administer antidiarrheal medications, as ordered
   d. Assess nutritional status and administer nutritional supplements, as ordered
   e. Teach the patient and family about the possible causes of diarrhea and measures to control it
   f. Explain the importance of a low-residue, high-protein diet to decrease GI motility
   g. Instruct the patient to avoid foods that irritate or stimulate the GI tract, such as coffee, tea, and spicy, very hot, or very cold foods
   h. Increase the patient's daily fluid intake to at least 3000 ml (unless contraindicated) to replace lost fluids and prevent dehydration

     i. Encourage increased consumption of foods high in potassium to replace potassium lost in diarrhea; monitor serum potassium levels for hypokalemia

     j. Instruct the patient to report continued diarrhea to the nurse or physician

     k. Provide skin care for the perianal area; e.g., cleanse skin after each bowel movement, provide sitz baths, and apply lotion

F. Fatigue

1. General information

    a. Fatigue refers to a general feeling of physical or emotional exhaustion and lack of energy needed to respond to stimuli

    b. In fatigue states, energy expenditures exceed metabolic resources, resulting in nutritional depletion

    c. Possible cancer- and cancer treatment-related causes include increased metabolic needs resulting from tumor growth, accumulation of waste products secondary to cancer treatment or cancer-related cellular destruction, anemia resulting from inadequate nutritional intake, decreased nutritional intake related to nausea and vomiting from chemotherapy, chronic pain, and psychological disturbances that deplete emotional and metabolic resources

2. Assessment findings

    a. Anemia, marked by decreased hemoglobin and hematocrit levels

    b. Altered sleep patterns

    c. Altered life-style

    d. Altered emotional state, such as anxiety or depression

    e. Increased physiologic or psychological stress

    f. Decreased nutritional intake; altered nutritional status

    g. Pain

    h. Decreased mobility

    i. Advanced disease

3. Nursing interventions

    a. Teach the patient and family about possible causes of fatigue, and explain that fatigue should be only temporary

    b. Encourage the patient to discuss any feelings or anxieties that may be causing emotional stress

    c. Help the patient develop coping skills to alleviate emotional stress

    d. Help the patient obtain information that can help mitigate stress-producing situations, such as details about scheduled chemotherapy

    e. Take appropriate measures to help the patient maintain adequate patterns of sleep, rest, and exercise

    f. Instruct the patient to pace his activities and schedule adequate rest periods to minimize physical fatigue

    g. Encourage the patient to seek help with child care, housework, and other demanding activities when needed

    h. Instruct the patient to drink at least 3000 ml of fluid daily (unless contraindicated) to promote excretion of tumor waste products

    i. Administer analgesics, as ordered, to help pain control

    j. Transfuse packed red blood cells, as ordered, to improve erythrocyte count

G. Nausea and vomiting

1. General information
   a. Nausea is a distressing sensation of the urge to vomit
   b. Vomiting is the forceful expulsion of GI tract contents through the espohagus and out of the mouth
   c. The mechanism of nausea and vomiting is unknown, but it appears to involve stimulation of the true vomiting center by the chemoreceptor trigger zone (CTZ), the cerebral cortex, the hypothalamus, and mid-brain sympathetic visceral, vagal visceral, and vestibulocerebellar afferent pathways
   d. Possible cancer- and cancer treatment-related causes include stimulation of the CTZ by tumor byproducts, obstruction of the GI tract by a tumor, and adverse reactions to RT or chemotherapy
   e. Exposure to noxious odors often exacerbates nausea and vomiting
2. Assessment findings
   a. History of nausea and vomiting following cancer treatment
   b. Fluid and electrolyte imbalance
   c. Psychological factors, such as anxiety or anticipatory nausea and vomiting
   d. Excessive salivation
3. Nursing interventions
   a. Assess for and report abdominal distention or abnormal bowel sounds
   b. Monitor hydration status, and replace fluids and electrolytes, as ordered
   c. Position the patient on his side to prevent aspiration of vomitus
   d. Provide comfort measures; e.g., wash the patient's face with a cool cloth and have him rinse his mouth frequently
   e. Administer antiemetics, as ordered
   f. Instruct the patient to move and change position slowly
   g. Teach the patient relaxation and distraction techniques
   h. Encourage the patient to get adequate rest
   i. Encourage the patient to avoid exposure to noxious odors
   j. Instruct the patient and family to call the physician if vomiting persists without relief

H. Neutropenia

1. General information
   a. Neutropenia refers to an abnormally low level of neutrophils (a type of white blood cell) in the blood
   b. Possible cancer- and cancer treatment-related causes include RT- or chemotherapy-induced bone marrow suppression; tumor infiltration of bone marrow; and primary bone marrow disease, such as leukemia

    c. Neutropenia may predispose a patient to infection as a result of a reduced phagocytic ability in neutrophils, macrophages, and reticulum cells and compromised specific and nonspecific defense mechanisms

2. Assessment findings
   a. Leukopenia (white blood cell count <5,000 cells/mm³)
   b. Granulocytopenia (granulocyte count <1500 cells/mm³)
   c. Fever (concomitant use of corticosteroids may mask fever response)
   d. Signs and symptoms of infection, such as chills, tachycardia, tachypnea, inflammation, malaise, irritability, and restlessness

3. Nursing interventions
   a. Wash hands often while providing patient care to minimize risk of infection transmission
   b. Use aseptic technique for invasive procedures such as starting I.V. lines, catheterization, injections, and wound care to prevent infection
   c. Culture possible sources of infection, as ordered; sources may include wounds, urine, sputum, or blood
   d. Reduce doses of immunosuppressive medications, such as steroids or anti-inflammatory agents, as ordered
   e. Provide the patient with a private room to minimize the risk of infection transmission from other patients
   f. Ensure disinfection of walls and floors before patient occupies the room to minimize exposure to possible contaminants
   g. Provide a laminar air flow room, if necessary and available
   h. As ordered, place the patient in protective or reverse isolation for severe leukopenia (leukocyte count <1,000 cells/mm³) or granulocytopenia (granulocyte count <500 cells/mm³); use is controversial
   i. Require hand washing and wearing of gown, gloves, and mask for all staff and visitors entering the patient's room to minimize the risk of infection transmission
   j. Require the patient to wear a gown and mask when leaving the room to minimize exposure to contaminants
   k. Provide a low bacterial-level diet to minimize risk of infection
   l. Always use sterilized, disinfected instruments for any procedures to prevent infection transmission
   m. Administer antipyretics, as ordered, to reduce fever; may be needed for patients with temperatures of 100.4° F. (38° C.) and above
   n. Administer granulocyte infusions, as ordered, to elevate serum granulocyte level
   o. Institute measures to control temperature and reduce risk of infection, such as changing dressings often or administering antibiotics as ordered
   p. Teach the patient and family to recognize potential causes of infection
   q. Instruct them to promptly report any signs and symptoms of infection

I. Pain

1. General information
   a. Pain is a subjective sensation of discomfort or distress caused by noxious stimulation of nerve endings

b. Factors affecting a patient's pain response include perception of the pain, anxiety level, personal and cultural attitudes towards pain, and past experiences with pain

c. Possible cancer- and cancer treatment-related causes of pain include infiltration, compression, distention, inflammation, occlusion, or obstruction of tissues, nerves, or blood vessels by a tumor, and fibrosis secondary to RT or surgery that results in compression of tissues and nerves

2. Assessment findings
   a. Subjective reports of pain
   b. Crying
   c. Facial grimacing and writhing movements
   d. Holding or splinting painful area
   e. History of insufficient use of pain medications
   f. Inflammation
   g. Tachycardia
   h. Elevated blood pressure
   i. Alert and aroused mental state indicative of the "flight or fight" reaction
   j. Ulcerations
   k. Stomatitis

3. Nursing interventions
   a. Assess the patient's complaints of pain
   b. Always believe the patient's claims of pain and discomfort
   c. Assess for objective signs of pain, such as facial grimacing or holding the painful body part or area
   d. Evaluate the location, onset, and duration of pain
   e. Ask the patient to rate the pain's intensity on a numerical scale of 0 to 10, with 0 signifying no pain and 10 signifying the most intense pain imaginable; teach the patient to use this rating scale when describing pain to other health professionals
   f. Assess for aggravating and alleviating factors
   g. Teach the patient and family about the causes of the patient's pain
   h. Ask about the patient's previous experiences with pain and pain control
   i. Assess the patient's beliefs and attitudes about pain, such as the perceived relationship between pain and cancer
   j. Assess any social and cultural influences on the patient's perception of pain
   k. Evaluate how the patient and family respond to the pain
   l. Evaluate the effects of pain on the patient's life-style. Effects may include anxiety, depression, fear, immobility, isolation, substance abuse, use of pain for secondary gain, and mistrust of health care professionals
   m. Assess the patient's expectations of pain relief measures, and reassure him that multiple methods of pain relief are available and will be tried
   n. Regularly provide pain relief measures, as appropriate
   o. Discuss the various narcotic and nonnarcotic medications available to control pain

p. Instruct the patient to take medications on a regular schedule to prevent pain, rather than only after the pain becomes intense

q. Teach the patient to have prescriptions refilled before the on-hand supply of medication becomes exhausted

r. Explain and encourage the use of noninvasive methods of pain control, such as relaxation techniques, guided imagery, distraction, transcutaneous electrical nerve stimulation (TENS), acupressure, massage, and hot or cold stimuli

s. Explain invasive methods of pain control, such as acupuncture, nerve blocks, and neurosurgery (rhizotomy, cordotomy)

J. Stomatitis and mucositis

1. General information

a. Stomatitis is an inflammation of the oral mucosa; mucositis, an inflammation of mucous membranes

b. Possible cancer- and cancer treatment-related causes include tumor infiltration of the mucous membranes and adverse effects of RT or chemotherapy

c. The epithelial lining of the oral cavity and mucous membranes is replaced about every 7 days; such a rapid turnover of cells makes this region highly vulnerable to the adverse effects of cancer treatments

2. Assessment findings

a. Mild erythema, edema, and tenderness

b. Dryness and mild burning sensation in mouth and throat

c. White layer of fibrinous exudate

d. Altered or inhibited taste sensation

e. White "cottage cheese" patches (caused by candidiasis, a common fungal infection)

f. Painful vesicles (caused by herpes simplex, the most common viral infection); these vesicles rupture within 6 to 12 hours and become encrusted with dried exudate

g. Creamy-white, nonpurulent, raised areas with red bases (caused by gram-negative bacterial infections)

h. Raised, yellow-brown, wart-like plaques (caused by gram-positive bacterial infections)

3. Nursing interventions

a. Assess the oral cavity twice a day or more

b. Instruct the patient to perform a complete oral hygiene regimen after each meal and at bedtime to prevent stomatitis—including flossing and brushing, using a nonabrasive dentifrice (or baking soda and saline solution, hydrogen peroxide and saline or water solution, or baking soda and water) or removing and cleaning dentures

c. Advise the patient to use petroleum jelly or lip balm to keep lips moist and prevent added oral discomfort

d. Encourage the patient to drink 3000 ml of fluid each day to prevent excessive mucous membrane dryness and dehydration

    e. Instruct the patient to prevent mucosal trauma and irritation by avoiding alcohol, spices, and very hot or very cold foods

    f. Administer topical or systemic analgesics, as ordered

    g. Apply a protective topical substance, such as kaolin-containing substances, as necessary

    h. Encourage the patient to maintain a balanced nutritional intake to prevent malnutrition and speed healing

    i. As ordered, administer medications to control infection

    j. Promptly report any signs and symptoms of infection

    k. Assist the patient with oral care; severe stomatitis requires care every 2 hours

    l. If stomatitis occurs, discontinue the patient's use of irritants, such as dentures, dental floss, and toothbrush

K. Thrombocytopenia

1. General information

    a. Thrombocytopenia is a hematologic disorder involving a reduction in the number of circulating platelets, which can predispose a patient to hemorrhagic disorders

    b. Possible cancer- and cancer treatment-related causes include primary disease of the bone marrow, such as leukemia; secondary disease of the bone marrow, such as tumor infiltration; and RT- or chemotherapy-induced bone marrow suppression

2. Assessment findings

    a. Petechiae

    b. Ecchymoses

    c. Platelet count $<100,000/mm^3$

    d. Bleeding from operative or invasive procedure sites or body orifices

    e. Hematuria

    f. Hematochezia

    g. Hematemesis

    h. Increased menstrual flow

3. Nursing interventions

    a. Assess laboratory values, especially platelet count, hemoglobin, and hematocrit

    b. Observe for any frank bleeding

    c. Assess drainage from GI tubes and wound sites for color, consistency, and presence of occult blood (e.g., "coffee grounds" in nasogastric suction drainage)

    d. Assess for occult blood in stool, urine, emesis, and sputum

    e. Monitor menstrual pad count and saturation level

    f. Avoid administering medications that can alter platelet function, such as aspirin

    g. Minimize skin trauma by coordinating venipunctures to decrease frequency and by avoiding parenteral injections

    h. Administer platelet infusions, as ordered

i. Institute bleeding precautions if platelet count is <50,000/mm³
j. Advise the patient to use an electric razor and a soft-bristle toothbrush and to avoid dental floss, to minimize the risk of bleeding
k. Discuss a bowel training program to prevent constipation and avoid straining during defecation, which increases intracranial pressure and may possibly cause intracerebral bleeding
l. Instruct the patient to avoid using enemas, suppositories, and rectal thermometers, to prevent rectal mucosal trauma and bleeding
m. Humidify room air and teach the patient to blow nose gently to minimize nasal mucosal trauma
n. Instruct the patient to avoid strenuous or risky activities, to minimize the risk of trauma that could precipitate bleeding
o. Encourage the female patient to use a lubricant during intercourse to minimize vaginal mucosal irritation or trauma. Instruct her to avoid intercourse if her platelet count is <50,000/mm³
p. Instruct the patient to apply pressure to a puncture site for 5 minutes following an injection, to help ensure adequate clotting
q. Encourage the patient to eat a high-protein diet to promote megakaryocyte formation

Points to Remember

Cancer patients commonly experience problems resulting from the disease itself, its treatment, or the adverse effects of treatment.

Common problems include alopecia, nausea and vomiting, diarrhea, neutropenia, and anemia.

Patient and family education is essential in dealing successfully with these problems.

Glossary

Hematemesis—blood in vomitus

Hematuria—blood in urine

Megakaryocyte—large bone marrow cell essential for platelet production

Myelosuppression—inhibited bone marrow function resulting in decreased blood cell and platelet production

Phagocytic—ability to surround, engulf, and digest microorganisms and cellular debris

Nursing Management of Patient and Family Psychosocial Needs

Learning Objectives
After studying this section, the reader should be able to:

• Identify the illness phases of cancer care.

• Describe significant aspects of each phase.

• Identify four common stressors associated with each phase.

• Discuss possible psychosocial nursing interventions for each phase.

VI. Nursing Management of Patient and Family Psychosocial Needs

A. Introduction

1. A diagnosis of cancer is a frightening and stress-producing event for a patient and family
2. The patient and family may experience stressors related to their perception of the disease and its treatment
3. Patients and family members cope with stressors differently
4. Factors affecting a patient's coping ability include:
   a. Perception of illness and treatment
   b. Previous experience with stressors
   c. Timing of the stressor
   d. Patient's stage in life
   e. Level of family support
   f. Cultural beliefs
   g. Societal attitudes
5. Acute exacerbation of disease may pose a crisis; the patient and family must adapt or alter their coping mechanisms
6. Psychosocial needs of a patient and family depend on illness phase
7. Illness phases include:
   a. Acute phase: diagnosis
   b. Chronic phase: during treatment
   c. Chronic phase: after successful treatment when disease is in remission
   d. Chronic phase: continued treatment when initial treatment proves unsuccessful and disease recurs
   e. Terminal phase
   f. Bereavement phase

B. Acute phase

1. General information
   a. The acute phase refers to the period beginning when cancer is first suspected and ending when diagnosis confirms cancer and a treatment plan is established
   b. This phase encompasses the initial disclosure of diagnosis to the patient and the patient's response
   c. Psychosocial implications involve the patient's reaction to the diagnosis and the impact of diagnosis on the patient's relationships with family, friends, neighbors, and co-workers
   d. The manner in which the diagnosis is communicated to the patient and family can enhance or damage their trust in health care professionals
   e. Disclosing a diagnosis to a patient does not increase the likelihood that he will commit suicide
   f. Initial responses to a diagnosis vary among patients; may be adaptive or maladaptive
   g. Adaptive responses include grief, depression, and anger; maladaptive responses include self-destructive behavior, extreme emotional distress, and noncompliance

    h. The significance that a patient attaches to a diagnosis of cancer varies, depending on the patient's knowledge of cancer, previous experience with cancer, patient's locus of control (internal or external), type of cancer and body area involved, and perception of effect on daily life and ability to achieve future goals

2. Common stressors
   a. Fear of the unknown
   b. Fear of pain and suffering
   c. Fear of death
   d. Fear of disfigurement
   e. Fear of doctors, tests, and hospitals
   f. Fear of income loss
   g. Fear of disability
   h. Fear of isolation, separation from loved ones
   i. Fear of losing control
   j. Fear of family's response

3. Nursing interventions
   a. Help the health care team choose an appropriate time to discuss the diagnosis with the patient
   b. Help determine who should be present to provide support when diagnosis is disclosed to the patient
   c. Help the patient differentiate accurate and inaccurate information about disease and diagnosis
   d. Encourage the patient to explore possible reasons why he developed cancer, but explain that the exact cause remains unknown
   e. Support the patient's reaction to diagnosis
   f. Identify how the patient and family respond to diagnosis
   g. Support adaptive coping responses
   h. Identify maladaptive responses
   i. Help the patient and family replace maladaptive behavior with adaptive behavior
   j. Help the patient identify the significance of the cancer type or body part affected
   k. Help the patient cope with the threat of losing a body part, losing the function of a body part, or disfigurement
   l. Discuss changes in life-style that may be necessary
   m. Help the patient adapt to changes in life-style
   n. Encourage family to accompany the patient to treatments
   o. Encourage the patient and family to discuss their feelings candidly
   p. Help the the patient understand his family's response to the diagnosis; discuss the reasons for their response
   q. Help the patient anticipate responses for inquiries about his condition
   r. Encourage the patient and family to initiate conversations about the disease, its treatment, and related topics
   s. Help the patient and spouse find ways to discuss illness with children
   t. Refer the patient and family to support groups and organizations

C. Chronic phase: during treatment
1. General information
    a. This phase refers to the period of initial treatment when the patient must live with the disease and treatment
    b. Patient and family emotional responses are primarily influenced by the progression of disease and any adverse effects of treatment
2. Common stressors
    a. Treatment regimen
    b. Adverse effects of treatment
    c. Adverse effects of disease
    d. Management of adverse effects
    e. Disease and treatment effects on personal relationships
    f. Impact of medical expenses on personal finances
    g. Changes in self-image
    h. Changes in body function
    i. Changes in sexual function
    j. Changes in sexual identity
    k. Worry about transportation to and from treatments
    l. Worry about impact of disease and treatment on family's life-style
3. Nursing interventions
    a. Teach the patient and family about treatments and possible adverse effects
    b. Help the patient manage adverse effects
    c. Help family and friends find ways to support the patient
    d. Support the patient's reaction to diagnosis
    e. Support adaptive coping behaviors
    f. Refer the patient to multidisciplinary health care team members, such as a psychologist or chaplain, when needed
    g. Refer the patient to a social worker for financial assistance as necessary
    h. Encourage the patient and family to discuss their feelings candidly
    i. Discuss the effects of treatment on the patient's self-image
    j. Help the patient adapt to changes in body function resulting from such procedures as colostomy or tracheostomy
    k. Teach the patient how to use prostheses, wigs, cosmetics, and similar items to make physical changes less noticeable
    l. Help the patient decide who to tell about changes in body function and when to tell them
    m. Assess the patient's sexual function
    n. Inform the patient and spouse that the patient's condition may necessitate alternative methods of sexual expression
    o. Teach the patient how reconstructive surgery may improve function or appearance

D. Chronic phase: after treatment (survivorship)
1. General information
    a. This phase refers to the period following initial treatment; characterized by regular follow-up visits with physician

      b. In this phase, disease is in remission but it is too early to presume the patient is cured

2. Common stressors
   a. Fear of disease recurrence
   b. Adjustment to a social network aware of the patient's disease
   c. Inability to return to previous occupation or to adjust to work load
   d. Difficulty in changing jobs because of diagnosis
   e. Adjustment to altered body function, possibly including altered sexual function
   f. Coping with residual effects of treatment, such as chronic pain or alopecia
   g. Management of medical expenses
   h. Adjustment to a family that has learned to function without the patient
   i. Coping with periodic diagnostic tests for disease recurrence

3. Nursing interventions
   a. Encourage the patient and family to openly discuss any fears they have about terminating treatment and the possibility of disease recurrence
   b. Discuss the possibility of disease recurrence
   c. Help the patient develop methods of coping with fear
   d. Discuss the patient's ability to work, to return to previous occupation, or to change jobs
   e. Refer the patient to a social worker for financial assistance and job counseling
   f. Discuss the potential difficulties of re-entering a social network with the patient
   g. Help the patient develop methods of coping with anticipated social encounters
   h. Initiate discussions about the patient's altered body functions and their impact on sexuality
   i. Help the patient find and adapt alternate methods of functioning
   j. Help the patient manage chronic symptoms to minimize their effects on life-style

E. Chronic phase: continued treatment

1. General information
   a. This phase refers to the period following initial treatment marked by residual disease or tumor recurrence and extending until the patient becomes terminal
   b. Patient and family emotional responses are strongly influenced by treatment goals, such as cure or palliation, and by any adverse effects of treatment

2. Common stressors
   a. Fear of death
   b. Fear of further pain and suffering
   c. Fear of disfigurement and disability
   d. Fear of financial loss

      e. Fear of isolation, abandonment by family and health care personnel

      f. Fear of losing control

      g. Fear of dependency

      h. Fear of family's response

      i. Fear of treatment and its adverse effects

3. Nursing interventions

      a. Help the health care team choose an appropriate time to discuss disease recurrence or further treatment with the patient

      b. Allow the patient to express feelings about disease recurrence

      c. Support adaptive coping behaviors

      d. Encourage open communication between the patient and family

      e. Help the patient with preparations for further treatment, such as planning time away from work and arranging transportation to treatments

      f. Teach the patient and family about the treatment plan and possible adverse effects

      g. Discuss treatment rationale and goals, such as disease palliation or control

      h. Manage adverse effects of treatment with the patient

      i. Allow expressions of grief and loss by the patient and family as the patient's disability and dependency increase

      j. Refer the patient and family to support personnel, such as visiting nurses or home health aides, for continuing patient care

F. Terminal phase

1. General information

      a. This phase refers to the period when the patient and family realize cure is not possible and death is inevitable

      b. Response of the patient and family to inevitable death depends on their existing coping methods

      c. A terminal patient often loses his sense of social value

      d. The nurse's perception of a patient's social value affects the quality of care she provides

      e. The dying trajectory assigned to a patient can influence the nurse's perception of the patient's illness and consequently the care she provides

      f. According to Avery Weisman, each dying patient needs to experience an appropriate death which involves symptom relief; comfort and support; a calm emotional environment; open, informative communication; relinquishing control of events; preserving token functions of life; and resolving or redefining any remaining problems

      g. Dying patients and their families may go through a series of distinct stages as death nears; described in theories of E.K. Ross, B. Giaquinta, and M. Pattison

      h. The experience of dying is unique for each terminal patient and must viewed that way by health care personnel; forcing a patient to pass through the sequential stages is inappropriate

2. Common stressors
    a. Physical decline
    b. Anxiety about death
    c. Fear of abandonment
    d. Fear of pain
    e. Loss of control
    f. Loss of ability to achieve goals
    g. Loss of social worth
    h. Loss of identity
    i. Loss of relationships with people and things, such as family home or a valued possession
3. Nursing interventions
    a. Be aware that unconsciously assigning decreased social value to a dying patient may affect nursing care
    b. Help the patient realize his value as an individual and as a family member
    c. Help the patient understand that dying does not affect his identity and self-worth
    d. Discuss past roles, accomplishments, and relationships with the patient
    e. Recognize the patient's process of dying; do not impose personal perceptions of dying on the patient
    f. Recognize that patients respond uniquely to dying
    g. Do not force the patient and family to pass through stages of dying in sequence; respond uniquely to each terminal patient and family
    h. Provide the patient with emotional support to lessen the impact of losses experienced during the terminal phase
    i. Allow the patient to grieve over losses
    j. Encourage activities that let the patient exercise control
    k. Help the patient and family set realistically attainable goals
    l. Assess each family member's ability to cope with the dying process
    m. Include family members in plan of care
    n. Encourage family members to care for their personal needs and not to exhaust themselves addressing the patient's needs
    o. Encourage family members to express their feelings
    p. Encourage family members to seek emotional support for their own needs
    q. Reassure family that guilt and resentment are common reactions
    r. Accept family members' responses to the dying patient
    s. Encourage family members who can provide patient support to fill in when other family members cannot
    t. Encourage communication between the patient and family members
    u. Reassure family members that anticipatory grieving is a normal, adaptive behavior

G. Bereavement phase
1. General information
   a. This phase refers to the period following death of a patient when family members resolve feelings about the patient's death; length of time varies greatly
   b. Mourning rituals vary among cultures; all seek to validate the death, provide guidelines for acceptable behavior, reaffirm group unity, emphasize importance of the deceased, lessen feelings of guilt, provide emotional support, and provide an outlet for emotions
   c. American culture venerates the dead and permits women more emotional expressions of grief than men
   d. Bereaved persons are more likely to experience illness and death than the general population
   e. Mortality rate for surviving spouses is highest during 6 months following death of spouse; rate then drops to mortality rate of the general population
   f. Risk of dying is greater for widowers than widows, especially young widowers
   g. Death of a parent may adversely affect a child's social and emotional development
2. Grief
   a. Grief, as defined by Erich Lindemann (1944), is a syndrome with five major symptoms: somatic distress, hostile reactions, preoccupation with image of the deceased, guilt, and loss of patterns of conduct
   b. It also maybe defined as a reactive depression that rarely requires psychiatric intervention
   c. Three phases of grief include shock and disbelief, developing awareness, and resolution
   d. Shock and disbelief protects individuals from emotional pain
   e. Developing awareness means realizing and accepting the loss
   f. The first two phases may occur over minutes, days, or months
   g. Resolution involves restructuring one's life around the loss, a process that typically takes a year
3. Factors affecting bereavement
   a. Amount of preparation for the patient's death
   b. Relationship between the terminal patient and survivors
   c. Family structure of the survivors
   d. Quality of the marital or personal relationship
   e. Dying process, such as amount of suffering and disfigurement experienced by the patient
   f. Ability to express emotions
   g. Previous exposure to death
   h. Use of anticipatory grieving
4. Nursing interventions
   a. Assess family's past coping ability

    b. Provide a private area where family members can be informed of the patient's death

    c. Arrange access to a telephone for family members so they can notify others

    d. Maintain your composure

    e. Stay with family members if asked or needed

    f. Let family members perform necessary closure activities, such as crying over, touching, or caressing the deceased

    g. Explain the procedures for transferring the body to a funeral home

    h. Inform the family of feelings and reactions they may experience during bereavement

    i. Explain that grieving may continue for a year

    j. Counsel the bereaved not to make major changes in their lives during the grieving period

    k. Stress the importance of having someone to share feelings with and confide in

    l. Provide support for the bereaved in the weeks following the patient's death by phoning or writing

Points to Remember

Diagnosis of cancer causes a life crisis for a patient and family during the acute phase of illness.

During the chronic phase of illness, patient and family emotional responses are governed primarily by progress of the disease and adverse effects experienced by the patient.

The patient's perception of his social value may effect his ability to cope with the terminal phase of cancer.

A person usually requires a year to resolve grief caused by the death of a loved one.

Appropriate responses by health care professionals during each phase of illness may facilitate the patient's and family's ability to cope.

Glossary

Bereavement—state of suffering over the death of a loved one

Coping—adaptation to stress

Crisis—state encountered when usual problem-solving methods prove ineffective

Dying trajectory—perceived course of dying consciously or unconsciously assigned to a patient

Grief—emotional response to loss involving physical and emotional distress

Mourning—expressions of grief following the death of a loved one

Cancer of the Skin

Learning Objectives

After studying this section, the reader should be able to:

• Discuss the epidemiology and risk factors for skin cancers.

• List possible clinical manifestations of each cancer.

• Discuss common routes of dissemination for each cancer.

• Identify several medical and surgical interventions for each cancer.

• Discuss nursing interventions for patients undergoing treatment for skin cancer.

VII. Cancer of the Skin

A. Introduction
1. Cancers of the skin—the most common type of cancer—threaten not only a patient's health but also his self-image by causing disfiguring lesions
2. Primary goals of intervention are prevention and early detection

B. Malignant melanomas
1. General information
   a. Most melanomas form near the basal lamina of the skin
   b. Melanomas can occur virtually anywhere on the body surface
   c. *Superficial spreading melanomas* (SSM) represent about 70% of all melanomas. Most common in women, these melanomas grow radially, then vertically, and often occur on the back
   d. *Nodular melanomas* (NM) comprise 15% of all melanomas. Most common in men, these melanomas have rapid vertical growth and may extend deep into the skin structure
   e. *Lentigo maligna melanomas* (LMM) typically occur on the face and neck. These slow-growing melanomas extend laterally before vertical growth occurs
   f. *Acral-lentiginous melanomas* (ALM) rarely occur and often are not listed as a classification of malignant melanomas
2. Epidemiology
   a. Incidence is rising; currently, 9 of every 100,000 patients examined for malignant melanomas are diagnosed positive
   b. Men and women are at equal risk for developing malignant melanomas; however, some types occur more often in one sex than the other
   c. Peak incidence occurs between ages 50 and 70
   d. Incidence is lowest in blacks and other dark-skinned persons
3. Risk factors
   a. Chronic exposure to ultraviolet light, typically from unprotected overexposure to sunlight
   b. History of acquired and dysplastic nevi
   c. Dysplastic nevus syndrome
   d. Family history of malignant melanomas
4. Clinical manifestations
   a. SSM: irregularly shaped lesion that ulcerates and bleeds as it grows
   b. NM: blue-black lesion with distinct borders
   c. LMM: freckle-like lesion with complex color patterns and vertical penetration
   d. ALM: irregularly shaped blue-black lesion of variable size; smooth or ulcerated, and raised or flat
5. Diagnostic procedures
   a. Excisional biopsy
   b. Incisional biopsy

6. Staging
   a. Clark's level of staging is most often used (may also use tumor, node, metastasis [TNM] staging system); most important criteria is the depth of skin penetration
   b. Procedures used in staging may include complete blood count, blood chemistries, chest X-ray, guaiac testing of stool, ECG, biopsy of enlarged lymph nodes, and radioisotopic scan of bone, brain, or liver
7. Natural progression of disease
   a. Routes of metastasis include local, radial, vertical, or horizontal invasion of skin; invasion of dermal lymphatic vessels, resulting in new regional satellite lesions; and invasion of lymphatic and vascular systems, resulting in local, regional, and distant lymph node involvement
   b. Sites of metastasis include local and deep satellites on skin; local, regional, and distant lymph nodes; and the liver, lungs, and brain
   c. Prognosis depends on depth of invasion, presence of satellite lesions, and extension of disease to lymph nodes; 5-year survival rate ranges from 100% for Stage I disease to 15% for Stage V disease
8. Nursing interventions for screening, detection, and prevention
   a. Instruct the patient to avoid prolonged exposure to sunlight and to especially avoid excessive tanning and sunburn
   b. Tell the patient to apply a topical sunscreen or sunblock with a protection factor greater than 10 before prolonged exposure to sunlight, and to reapply it every 2 to 3 hours during exposure
   c. Advise the patient to wear protective clothing if prolonged sun exposure is unavoidable
   d. Warn the patient to avoid ultraviolet light and X-ray treatments for skin conditions
   e. Instruct the patient to check skin for lesions once a month and to seek prompt medical attention for any suspicious lesions
9. Nursing interventions for psychosocial needs
   a. Encourage the patient to express feelings regarding diagnosis, treatment plan, and impact of disease on his life-style
   b. Encourage open communication between the patient and family
   c. Assess patient and family coping mechanisms
   d. Determine the availability of support resources, and help the patient gain access to appropriate resources
   e. Discuss any feelings of guilt the patient may have about a history of excessive unprotected sun exposure
   f. Assess the possible impact of surgery on the patient, especially potentially disfiguring surgery
10. Surgical interventions
    a. Curative surgery for malignant melanomas typically involves local excision of the primary tumor with wide margins
    b. Defects caused by excision may require skin grafts
    c. Prophylactic dissection of regional lymph nodes also may be performed

11. Nursing interventions for patients undergoing surgery
    a. Provide general nursing care measures applicable to all patients undergoing surgery (see Section II.B)
    b. Assess the viability of any skin grafts
    c. Assess donor sites for signs of bleeding and infection
    d. Perform donor and graft site care, as ordered
    e. Teach the patient and family proper wound care procedures, such as cleansing and dressing, as needed
    f. Explain that regular follow-up examinations are necessary to check for disease recurrence
12. Radiotherapeutic interventions
    a. Radiation therapy (RT) is not used as a primary or adjuvant treatment for malignant melanomas
    b. Its use in treating recurring disease is currently being studied
    c. RT may be used in palliative treatment of metastatic disease
13. Nursing interventions for patients receiving RT
    a. Provide general nursing care measures applicable to all patients receiving RT (see Section II.C)
    b. Encourage the patient to express feelings about the disease's progression and possible consequences
14. Chemotherapeutic interventions
    a. Chemotherapy used as an adjuvant to surgery does not improve survival rate
    b. It may be used to palliate symptoms
    c. Limb-perfusion chemotherapy using dacarbazine (DTIC) and nitrosoureas may minimize systemic toxicity; response rate is good
    d. Interferon is used to treat recurring or metastatic disese; response rate is 30%, and persons who respond have an increased survival rate
    e. Bacillus Calmette-Guérin and other immunotherapeutic agents have been used to treat malignant melanomas
15. Nursing interventions for patients receiving chemotherapy
    a. Provide general nursing care measures applicable to all patients receiving chemotherapy (see Section II.D)
    b. Teach the patient and family about limb-perfusion chemotherapy; discuss the logistics and rationale of this treatment
    c. Assess for signs and symptoms of bleeding from limb-perfusion injection site
    d. Evaluate circulation and function in the extremity used in limb-perfusion chemotherapy; report any signs and symptoms of reduced circulation or function

C. Nonmelanomas
1. General information
   a. Nonmelanomas include basal cell carcinomas (BCC) and squamous cell carcinomas (SCC)

      b. The most common type of BCC is nodular-ulcerated BCC, which typically occurs on the face

      c. SCCs include aggressive SCCs and Bowen's disease (carcinoma in situ)

2. Epidemiology

      a. Nonmelanomas are the most common type of cancer and the cancer most likely to entail other multiple primary occurrences (second cancers)

      b. Each year, 5 to 10 million patients are diagnosed as having nonmelanomas

      c. Nonmelanomas carry a very low mortality rate, accounting for less than 0.1% of all cancer deaths

3. Risk factors

      a. Prolonged, repeated exposure to ultraviolet radiation, typically from sunlight

      b. Chronic exposure to ionizing radiation

      c. Chronic exposure to arsenic

      d. Chronic exposure to petrochemicals, such as coal tar

      e. Genetic defect, such as xeroderma pigmentosum

      f. Immunodeficiency or immunosuppression

      g. History of chronic skin inflammation or trauma, such as fistula formation

      h. History of premalignant skin lesions or conditions, such as Bowen's disease, actinic or senile keratosis, and seborrheic keratosis

4. Clinical manifestations

      a. BCC: raised, hard, erythematous, centrally ulcerated, pearly lesions

      b. SCC (early): scaly, keratotic lesions with raised irregular borders; history of chronic ulceration

      c. SCC (late): exophytic, friable, chronically crusting lesions

5. Diagnostic procedures

      a. Excisional biopsy

      b. Incisional biopsy

6. Staging

      a. The TNM system of staging is used

      b. Procedures used to determine staging vary, depending on extent of lesions

7. Natural progression of disease

      a. Routes of metastasis include direct invasion (BCC) and through the hematologic and lymphatic systems (SCC)

      b. Sites of metastasis include the skin surface (BCC, although metastasis rarely occurs) and regional draining lymph nodes, distant lymph nodes, and distant organs (SCC)

      c. Prognosis: cure rate for BCC is 90% to 95%; for SCC, 70% to 80%

8. Nursing interventions for screening, detection, and prevention

      a. Instruct the patient to avoid prolonged exposure to sunlight and to especially avoid excessive tanning and sunburn

      b. Tell the patient to apply a topical sunscreen or sunblock with a protection factor greater than 10 before prolonged exposure to sunlight, and to reapply it every 2 to 3 hours during exposure

     c. Advise the patient to wear protective clothing if prolonged sun exposure is unavoidable

     d. Warn the patient to avoid ultraviolet light and X-ray treatments for skin conditions

     e. Instruct the patient to check skin for lesions once a month and to seek prompt medical attention for any suspicious lesions

9. Nursing interventions for psychosocial needs
   a. Encourage the patient to express feelings regarding diagnosis, treatment plan, and impact of disease on his life-style
   b. Encourage open communication between the patient and family
   c. Assess patient and family coping mechanisms
   d. Determine the availability of support resources, and help the patient gain access to appropriate resources
   e. Discuss any feelings of guilt the patient may have about a history of excessive unprotected sun exposure
   f. Assess the possible impact of surgery on the patient, especially potentially disfiguring surgery

10. Surgical interventions
    a. Surgical resection is the primary treatment for recurring disease
    b. Resection includes excision of sizeable margins of unaffected tissue to prevent recurrence
    c. Curettage may be used for superficial BCC
    d. Other surgical options include cryosurgery and laser surgery

11. Nursing interventions for patients undergoing surgery
    a. Provide general nursing care measures applicable for all patients undergoing surgery (see Section II.B)
    b. Teach the patient and family proper surgical site care, such as keeping the incision site or area of laser therapy dry
    c. Explain that regular follow-up examinations are necessary to check for disease recurrence

12. Radiotherapeutic interventions
    a. RT can effectively treat areas prone to surgical disfigurement, such as eyelids
    b. RT typically is limited to older patients because of the risks that possible radiation-induced cancer pose for younger patients

13. Nursing interventions for patients receiving RT for nonmelanomas are similar to those for any patient receiving RT (see Section II.C)

14. Chemotherapeutic interventions
    a. Topical 5-fluorouracil is effective in treating Bowen's disease
    b. Systemically administered chemotherapy may be used if surgery or RT fails to control advanced disease

15. Nursing interventions for patients receiving chemotherapy
    a. Provide general nursing care measures applicable to all patients receiving chemotherapy (see Section II.D)
    b. Teach the patient using 5-fluorouracil cream how to apply it properly. Even when used properly, it can cause skin irritation; improper use may cause tissue sloughing

Points to Remember

Nonmelanoma skin cancers are the most common type of cancer.

The incidence of skin cancer is rising, with excessive unprotected sun exposure the apparent cause.

Malignant melanomas require aggressive treatment with surgery and occasionally chemotherapy.

The most important criterion for determining the staging and prognosis of malignant melanomas is the depth of skin penetration.

Glossary

Actinic—relating to the visible and ultraviolet radiation that causes photochemical reactions, as in sunlight

Basal lamina—uppermost layer of the basement membrane, the deepest skin layer

Keratosis—skin condition characterized by excessive growth of the horny layer

Nevus—circumscribed malformation of the skin; may involve hyperpigmentation or increased vascularity

Pearly lesion—shiny, cloudy-white skin lesion

Cancer of the Head, Neck, and Chest

Learning Objectives

After studying this section, the reader should be able to:

- Discuss the epidemiology and risk factors for head, neck, and chest cancers.

- List possible clinical manifestations of each cancer.

- Identify several tests used to diagnose and stage each cancer.

- Discuss common routes of dissemination for each cancer.

- Identify several medical and surgical interventions for each cancer.

- Discuss nursing interventions for patients undergoing treatment for head, neck, or chest cancer.

VIII. Cancer of the Head, Neck, and Chest

A. Introduction

1. Because of their location, cancers of the head, neck, and chest threaten major anatomical structures and blood vessels
2. Bronchogenic (lung) cancer is the most prevalent primary cancer of the chest
3. Cigarette smoking is a major risk factor for head, neck, and chest cancers

B. Head and neck cancer

1. General information
   a. Cancer lesions typically occur concurrently in head and neck tissues, possibly as a result of simultaneous exposure to carcinogenic agents
   b. Most head and neck cancers (95%) are of squamous cell origin
   c. Most patients (80% to 90%) present with lesions 2 cm (¾″) or larger; 60% of patients present with advanced disease
   d. Incidence of second primary cancer is high; 5% of patients have second primary cancer at time of diagnosis
   e. Between 20% and 30% of patients with head and neck cancer will develop a second primary cancer after treatment for the initial cancer
   f. Patients who develop second primary cancers often experience immunosuppression, particularly suppressed T-cell function
2. Epidemiology
   a. Head and neck cancers account for 4% of all cancers diagnosed in men and 2% of all cancers diagnosed in women in the United States
   b. Head and neck cancers cause 2% of male cancer deaths and 1% of female cancer deaths in the United States
   c. Incidence is higher in lower socioeconomic groups
   d. Peak incidence occurs between ages 50 and 60, and again between ages 70 and 80
   e. Incidence of nasal pharynx, nasal cavity, and paranasal sinus cancer is higher in persons of Asian descent
3. Risk factors
   a. Excessive long-term alcohol consumption
   b. Cigarette smoking
   c. Combined use of alcohol and cigarettes (greatly increases risk)
   d. Use of chewing tobacco
   e. Dietary deficiency of vitamin A and retinoids
   f. Chronic exposure to wood dust, nickel compounds, nitrosamines, hydrocarbons, or asbestos
   g. Alterations in the oral cavity, nasal cavity, or paranasal sinuses, such as those caused by poor oral hygiene or dentition, prolonged focused irritation from dentures, syphilis, Plummer-Vinson syndrome, and Epstein-Barr virus infection
4. Clinical manifestations
   a. Leukoplakia
   b. Erythroplasia

    c. Palpable or visible tissue mass
    d. Ulceration
    e. Localized or referred pain
    f. Dysphagia
    g. Odynophagia
    h. Hoarseness
    i. Diplopia
    j. Cranial nerve palsy
    k. Nasal blockage or bleeding

5. Diagnostic tests
    a. Nasopharyngoscopy
    b. Laryngoscopy
    c. Esophagoscopy
    d. Brush biopsy cytology
    e. Biopsy

6. Staging
    a. The tumor, node, metastasis (TNM) system of staging is used
    b. Procedures used in staging may include head and neck xerography, barium swallow esophagography, sialography, blood chemistries, chest X-ray, head and neck X-rays, and head and neck tomography

7. Natural progression of disease
    a. Routes of metastasis include local extension, perineural spread, orderly progression through the lymphatic system, and hematogenous spread (late occurrence)
    b. Sites of metastasis include regional lymph nodes and adjacent structures, lungs, liver, and bone
    c. Prognosis: Cervical lymph node involvement in local or regional disease is a critical indicator. Undifferentiated tumors are more likely to metastasize to lymph nodes. Prognosis worsens as lymph node involvement increases, with most patients dying within 18 months of recurrence

8. Nursing interventions for screening, detection, and prevention
    a. Be aware of risk factors and signs and symptoms of head and neck cancers
    b. Explain to patients the rationale for limiting or eliminating alcohol and tobacco use
    c. Encourage patients with possible early symptoms of head and neck cancers to seek prompt medical attention

9. Nursing interventions for psychosocial needs
    a. Assess the patient's psychological response to diagnosis and the need for treatment
    b. Assess patient and family coping mechanisms
    c. Determine the availability of support resources, and help the patient gain access to appropriate resources
    d. Evaluate the patient's ability and willingness to comply with the treatment plan

     e. Assess the patient's fears about possible adverse effects of treatment, such as cosmetic defects, speech impairment, or impaired ability to eat

     f. Teach the patient and family about reconstructive surgery and rehabilitative therapy options

10. Surgical interventions

     a. Surgery is the preferred treatment modality for most head and neck cancers

     b. Radical surgery, used for curative treatment, involves en bloc resection of tumor, involved lymph nodes, and a wide margin of tumor-free tissue

     c. Cosmetic reconstruction requirements must be assessed before radical surgery

     d. Oral cavity and oropharynx cancers are treated with radical surgery, such as commando procedures, monobloc resection, or composite resection; involves en bloc removal of tumor, cervical lymph nodes, and part of the mandible, if necessary

     e. Radical neck dissection involves en bloc removal of tumor and sternocleidomastoid muscle, internal jugular vein, and cranial nerve XI (accessory)

     f. Modified radical neck dissection is used if cervical lymph nodes are negative upon clinical examination; postoperative radiation therapy (RT) is planned; neck involvement is minimal; or such structures as the cranial nerve XI or sternocleidomastoid muscle can be preserved

     g. Partial neck dissection involves partial resection of the lymph node chain

11. Nursing interventions for patients undergoing surgery

     a. Provide general nursing care measures applicable to all patients undergoing surgery (see Section II.B)

     b. Assess teeth, gingivae, and oral cavity, and evaluate ability to chew and swallow

     c. Teach the patient about the importance of good nutrition; provide supplements as necessary to improve nutritional status before surgery

     d. Refer the patient to an oral surgeon before surgery, if necessary, to plan future reconstructive surgery

     e. When surgery impairs speech, arrange for alternate methods of patient communication, such as pad and pencil or chalkboard

     f. As necessary, teach the patient and family about proper tracheostomy or laryngectomy care procedures

     g. After surgery, assess patency of airway or tracheostomy to prevent postoperative airway obstruction

     h. Suction the airway as necessary and encourage the patient to turn, cough, and deep-breathe regularly to remove secretions and maintain airway patency

     i. Assess for signs and symptoms of hemorrhage; carotid artery rupture can occur, especially if the carotid artery is exposed as a result of flap necrosis or continued tumor growth

     j. Assess for hematomas, especially beneath skin flaps, which can prevent flap adherence to underlying tissue and result in necrosis

      k. Assess patency of drainage tubes under skin flaps; prevent fluid accumulation to facilitate flap adherence to underlying tissue

      l. Elevate the head of the bed to facilitate swallowing and improve lymphatic and venous drainage

     m. Prevent torsion or tension on skin flaps or suture lines, which can cause wound separation or breakdown

      n. Provide or instruct the patient to perform meticulous oral hygiene four times a day, paying special attention to intra-oral suture lines; warn against using commercial mouthwashes, which can cause irritation

      o. Be aware that wound infection can cause orocutaneous or pharyngo-cutaneous fistula formation; administer antibiotics, as ordered, and give the patient nothing by mouth until fistula heals

      p. Assess for possible thoracic lymph duct leakage in inferior neck area (chyle leakage is white); may cease spontaneously or require surgery

      q. As ordered, provide nutritional support with enteral or parenteral supplements to promote wound healing

      r. Encourage early ambulation when possible to prevent thrombus formation; administer anticoagulants, as ordered, to immobile patients

      s. Assess for possible nerve injury; findings may include paresthesia, paralysis, shoulder droop, altered taste sensation, difficulty swallowing, or speech impediments

      t. As necessary, refer the patient to a speech therapist for language training, rehabilitative exercises, prosthesis fitting, or swallow training

12. Radiotherapeutic interventions

      a. The radiation field includes the area around the tumor and the first level of draining lymph nodes

      b. RT may be administered before resection to shrink large, bulky, fixed tumors

      c. However, preoperative RT may damage skin, lymphatic vessels, arteries, and veins, necessitating the use of skin flaps to close surgical sites

      d. Postoperative RT is currently in widespread use; involves administration of RT as an adjunctive therapy following surgical debulking of tumor and healing of healthy tissue

      e. Interstitial implants, which provide higher radiation doses than external beam RT, may be used to treat limited disease

13. Nursing interventions for patients receiving RT

      a. Provide general nursing care measures applicable to all patients receiving RT (see Section II.C)

      b. Inform the patient and family that xerostomia should improve over time, but may not disappear completely

      c. Also explain that acute mucositis should abate and the patient's sense of taste will return

      d. Evaluate skin for breakdown, especially in areas where carotid artery protection is reduced because of radical neck dissection

      e. Maintain adequate nutrition and hydration throughout treatment and the immediate posttreatment period

14. Chemotherapeutic interventions
    a. Chemotherapy may be used as an adjuvant treatment before surgery or RT
    b. It is used with RT to radiosensitize advanced local disease
    c. It may be used alone or in combination therapy for disseminated or recurrent disease
15. Nursing interventions for patients receiving chemotherapy for head and neck cancers involve general nursing care measures applicable for all patients receiving chemotherapy (see Section II.D)

C. Bronchogenic (lung) cancer
1. General information
   a. Most lung tumors (over 90%) arise from the bronchial epithelium
   b. Based on histology, bronchogenic cancer may be classified as small cell lung cancer or non-small cell lung cancer
   c. Small cell lung cancers include oat cell, hexagonal cell, lymphocytic, and spindle cell cancers
   d. Small cell lung cancers often occur near the mediastinum or hilus, are usually widespread when discovered, typically cause rapid patient deterioration, and often recur in local and distant sites
   e. Non-small cell lung cancers include squamous cell cancers, adenocarcinomas, epidermoid carcinomas, and large cell carcinomas
   f. Squamous cell cancers usually remain localized and recur locally following treatment; central tumors are more common than peripheral tumors
   g. Adenocarcinomas and large cell carcinomas most commonly occur in women and nonsmoking men
   h. The giant cell form of large cell carcinomas carries the poorest prognosis of all lung cancers
2. Epidemiology
   a. Lung cancer is the leading cause of cancer death in the United States, responsible for approximately 33% of all cancer deaths
   b. Peak incidence in men occurs between ages 50 and 60
   c. Incidence in women is rising rapidly; lung cancer became the leading cause of cancer death in women in 1985
   d. Incidence is highest in industrialized countries
   e. Squamous cell and epidermoid carcinomas are the most common lung cancers
3. Risk factors
   a. History of smoking (linked to 85% of all lung cancers); risk increases in proportion to duration and quantity of smoking, and decreases with cessation
   b. Chronic exposure to air pollution, particularly automobile and factory emissions and byproducts of sulfurous fuel combustion
   c. Chronic occupational exposure to asbestos, radiation, uranium, arsenic, coal distillates, iron oxide, or tar

     d. Genetic predisposition (according to some researchers)

     e. Exposure to multiple risk factors, such as smoking and working with asbestos, greatly increases risk

4. Clinical manifestations

     a. Cough

     b. Hemoptysis

     c. Dyspnea

     d. Wheezing

     e. Shoulder, arm, or chest pain

     f. Hoarseness

     g. Dysphagia

     h. Superior vena cava syndrome

5. Diagnostic tests

     a. Chest X-ray

     b. Lung tomography

     c. Bronchoscopy with brush biopsy

     d. Needle biopsy

     e. Cytologic examination of secretions or biopsied tissue

6. Staging

     a. The TNM staging system is used for lung cancer

     b. Procedures used in staging include chest X-ray, lung and hilar tomography, complete blood count and blood chemistry, ECG, transbronchial needle biopsy; mediastinoscopy; mediastinotomy; scalene node biopsy; liver, spleen, or bone scan; thoracentesis; computer tomography scan of chest or brain; and bone marrow biopsy

7. Natural progression of disease

     a. Routes of metastasis include direct extension, lymphatic spread, and hematogenous spread

     b. Sites of metastasis (determined by cell type and tumor location) include central hilar, mediastinal, peritracheal, supraclavicular, and cervical lymph nodes, liver, brain, bone, and adrenal glands

     c. Prognosis: Cure is rare because disease is usually advanced at diagnosis; 5-year survival rate is less than 10% for all stages and types of lung cancers

8. Nursing interventions for screening, detection, and prevention

     a. Explain that no accurate screening test for lung cancer exists

     b. Explain that the emphasis of nursing interventions is on prevention

     c. Explain the relationship between smoking and lung cancer and urge patients to stop smoking or to never start

     d. Refer patients who smoke to a smoking cessation program

     e. Provide a good role model for patients by not smoking

     f. Discuss possible ways to minimize exposure to occupational and environmental risk factors

9. Nursing interventions for psychosocial needs

     a. Encourage the patient to express feelings regarding diagnosis, treatment plan, and impact of disease on his life-style

      b. Discuss the possibility that treatment may cause respiratory disability, and discuss possible consequences of this disability

      c. Encourage open communication between the patient and family

      d. Assess patient and family coping mechanisms

      e. Determine the availability of support resources and help the patient gain access to appropriate resources

      f. Allow the patient or family members to discuss any feelings of guilt they may have about their history of cigarette smoking

      g. As necessary, refer the patient and family to multidisciplinary health care team members, such as a psychologist or chaplain

10. Surgical interventions

      a. Surgical resection is the preferred treatment for cure in patients with non-small cell Stage I or Stage II cancer

      b. Surgical interventions used include laser phototherapy (for small, local, superficial tumors accessible by bronchoscopy), lobectomy, sleeve lobectomy, wedge resection, pneumonectomy, and resection of the diaphragm or chest wall

11. Nursing interventions for patients undergoing surgery

      a. Provide general nursing care measures applicable to all patients undergoing surgery (see Section II.B)

      b. Assess respiratory function (including rate, presence of dyspnea, use of accessory muscles, and arterial blood gas results) for potential problems

      c. Assess for signs of bleeding, such as bloody sputum, tachycardia, or blood on dressing

      d. Assess for signs and symptoms of mediastinal shift after pneumonectomy, including restlessness, dyspnea, tachypnea, cyanosis, tachycardia, atrial dysrhythmias, shifted point of maximum impulse, and tracheal deviation from midline

      e. Evaluate chest tube function; maintain water seal and keep the device below the level of the patient's chest to promote drainage

      f. Promote optimal respiratory function; reposition the patient as needed and encourage regular turning, coughing, and deep breathing

      g. Provide pain control measures, including analgesics, as ordered

      h. Help the patient understand and adjust to life-style limitations imposed by impaired respiratory function

12. Radiotherapeutic interventions

      a. RT involves irradiation of areas surrounding tumors and metastatic sites

      b. Goals of RT include eradicating inoperable tumors; controlling local tumors, inoperable tumors, recurrences, pain, and bleeding; palliating superior vena cava syndrome, tracheal or bronchial obstruction, and symptoms of brain metastasis; and providing prophylactic treatment to prevent brain metastasis in small cell cancer

13. Nursing interventions for patients receiving RT

      a. Provide general nursing care measures applicable to all patients receiving RT (see Section II.C)

  b. Assess for esophagitis and dysphagia, and intervene as necessary to maintain optimal nutritional intake and hydration

  c. Assess respiratory function

  d. Promote optimum respiratory function by providing adequate hydration, encouraging diaphragmatic breathing, and using postural drainage to mobilize tenacious secretions. Keep in mind that coughing alone may not clear secretions

  e. Assess for skin reactions to RT, and take necessary steps to prevent skin breakdown

  f. Intervene as necessary to treat alopecia, otitis, transient central nervous system syndrome, and desquamation of portions of the ear following cranial RT

14. Chemotherapeutic interventions

  a. Chemotherapy is not indicated in early stage non-small cell lung cancer

  b. It effectively treats small cell lung cancers, with a response rate of 70% to 90%

  c. Chemotherapy is commonly used with cranial RT for improved survival rate in small cell lung cancer

  d. Combination chemotherapy improves non-small cell lung cancer response rate but not survival rate; response rate is 30% to 50%

  e. Commonly used antineoplastic agents include alkylating agents and vinca alkaloid combinations

15. Nursing interventions for patients receiving chemotherapy

  a. Provide general nursing care measures applicable to all patients receiving chemotherapy (see Section II.D)

  b. Monitor complete blood count and platelet count for abnormalities

  c. Assess for signs and symptoms of infection or bleeding

  d. Monitor for nausea and vomiting and intervene as necessary to help control it

  e. Assess nutritional status and administer supplements, as ordered; encourage increased protein and caloric intake

  f. Monitor intake and output and maintain hydration

  g. Promote good oral hygiene to prevent stomatitis

  h. Assess bowel elimination patterns for diarrhea or constipation and intervene as necessary for prevention or control

Points to Remember

Combined long-term use of alcohol and cigarettes substantially increases the risk of head and neck cancers.

The need for and extent of cosmetic reconstruction must be considered before treatment for head and neck cancers begins.

Treatment and rehabilitation for a patient with head and neck cancers require a multidisciplinary health care team approach.

Bronchogenic (lung) cancer is now the leading cause of cancer death in women.

Lung cancer usually carries a poor prognosis because of the difficulty of early detection and the typically advanced stage of disease at diagnosis.

Lung cancer is classified according to histology as small cell lung cancer or non-small cell lung cancer; each has specific treatments and prognoses.

Resection is the preferred treatment for early-stage non-small cell lung cancers.

Glossary

Chyle—liquid products of digestion (primarily absorbed fats) taken up by the small intestine and passed into the lymphatic system for transport to venous circulation at the thoracic duct in the neck

Cytology—the study of cell anatomy, physiology, pathology, and chemistry

Leukoplakia—precancerous, slowly developing change in a mucous membrane marked by thick, raised, sharply circumscribed white patches

Lobectomy—surgical procedure involving partial removal of a lung

Odynophagia—severe pain on swallowing

Scalene node—supraclavicular lymph node

Sialogram—diagnostic procedure involving x-ray of salivary gland and duct after injection of opaque media

Superior vena cava syndrome—obstruction of the superior vena cava that interferes with venous drainage from the head, upper thorax, and arms, leading to decreased venous return and increased venous pressure

Cancer of the GI Tract

Learning Objectives

After studying this section, the reader should be able to:

- Discuss the epidemiology and risk factors for GI tract cancers.

- List possible clinical manifestations of each cancer.

- Identify tests and studies used to diagnose and stage each cancer.

- Discuss common routes of dissemination for each cancer.

- Identify several medical and surgical interventions for each cancer.

- Discuss nursing interventions for patients undergoing treatment for GI tract cancer.

IX. Cancer of the GI Tract

A. **Introduction**
   1. Cancer effects the GI tract more often than any other organ system
   2. Onset of GI tract cancer typically is insidious, with clinical manifestations rarely appearing until disease is advanced
   3. Early detection and diagnosis of GI tract cancer is difficult because signs and symptoms often are misdiagnosed, self-treated, or ignored
   4. Surgery is the principal treatment modality used for GI tract cancer

B. **Esophageal cancer**
   1. General information
      a. The cause of esophageal cancer remains unknown
      b. Histologic cell types include squamous cell carcinoma (accounting for 98% of esophageal cancers) and adenocarcinomas (representing 2% of esophageal cancers)
      c. More than 40% of esophageal tumors develop in the lower thoracic esophagus
      d. Tumors may be exophytic, endophytic, or intramural
      e. Lesions usually ulcerate
      f. The tumor may encircle and thicken the esophageal wall or invade the submucosa, resulting in obstruction
   2. Epidemiology
      a. Esophageal cancer represents approximately 1% of all cancers diagnosed in the United States and accounts for about 2% of cancer deaths in the United States
      b. Mortality rate is higher in men than in women
      c. Persons between ages 50 and 70 are at highest risk, with average age of onset at 62
      d. On average, blacks develop esophageal cancer at a younger age than whites
      e. In the United States, incidence varies widely with geographical region (possibly indicating environmental influence)
   3. Risk factors
      a. Excessive alcohol consumption
      b. Excessive tobacco use
      c. Chronically poor oral hygiene
      d. History of malnutrition, vitamin deficiency, or anemia
      e. Chronic irritation from hiatal hernia, reflux esophagitis, diverticula, or Barrett's syndrome
      f. Ingestion of caustic agents, such as lye
      g. Chronic consumption of very hot foods or beverages
      h. Untreated achalasia
      i. Genetic conditions, such as tylosis
      j. Prolonged occupational exposure to ionizing radiation
      k. History of chronic exposure to chemicals, such as asbestos or nitrosamines

4. Clinical manifestations
   a. Indigestion (early symptom)
   b. Heartburn, substernal distress (early symptom)
   c. Loss of appetite
   d. Dysphagia (late symptom)
   e. Odynophagia (late symptom)
   f. Dehydration (late symptom)
   g. Malnutrition (late symptom)
   h. Anemia
   i. Hoarseness (resulting from laryngeal nerve paralysis)
   j. Hiccups
   k. Paralysis of arm or diaphragm (resulting from phrenic nerve involvement)
   l. Paresthesias (caused by brachial plexus involvement)
5. Diagnostic tests
   a. Barium swallow esophagography
   b. Endoscopic brush biopsy
6. Staging
   a. The tumor, node, metastasis (TNM) system is used to stage esophageal cancer
   b. Procedures used in staging include chest X-ray, complete blood count (CBC), blood chemistries, computer tomography (CT) scan of mediastinum and upper abdomen, and bone scan
7. Natural progression of disease
   a. Routes of metastasis include lymphatic spread, direct extension, and hematogenous spread
   b. Sites of metastasis include lymph nodes, lungs, liver, adrenal glands, bone, and kidneys
   c. Prognosis: 5-year survival rate is less than 10%
8. Nursing interventions for screening, detection, and prevention
   a. Keep in mind that no screening test for esophageal cancer exists
   b. Teach patients to avoid risk factors, such as excessive alcohol consumption and tobacco use
   c. Be aware of signs and symptoms of esophageal lesions
   d. Instruct the patient to seek prompt medical attention when symptoms appear
9. Nursing interventions for psychosocial needs
   a. Encourage the patient to express feelings about the diagnosis, treatment plan, and impact of the disease on his life-style
   b. Assess patient and family coping mechanisms
   c. Determine the availablity of support resources and help the patient gain access to appropriate resources
   d. Promote open communication between the patient and family
   e. Assess the patient's ability to cope with possible laryngectomy

      f. Refer the patient to multidisciplinary health care team members, such as social workers, speech therapists, or dietitians, as needed

      g. Refer the patient to appropriate support groups, such as a laryngectomy club

10. Surgical interventions

      a. Surgery for esophageal cancer is primarily aimed at cure, but is sometimes done to palliate symptoms

      b. Surgery is appropriate for resectable tumors with no involvement of contiguous structures

      c. Surgery is indicated in Stage I or Stage II disease with no distant metastasis

      d. Candidates for surgery must demonstrate adequate nutritional status and stable overall health

      e. Surgery for esophageal cancer carries a high postoperative mortality rate associated with pulmonary complications, anastomotic leakage, infection, and thromboembolism

      f. Partial cervical esophagectomy is indicated for cancer localized in the cervical esophagus; organ involvement necessitates laryngectomy or hypopharyngectomy

      g. Esophagectomy, used for lesions in the upper thoracic esophagus, requires reconstruction of esophagus using a section of colon or stomach or a prosthetic device

      h. Esophagectomy is rarely used, however, because in most patients with esophageal lesions, cancer is too far advanced for resection

      i. Esophagogastrectomy, used for lesions in the lower esophagus, also requires reconstruction of the esophagus involving elevation of the stomach with anastomosis to the remaining esophagus

11. Nursing interventions for patients undergoing surgery

      a. Teach the patient and family members about surgery, including probable extent of tissue removal and treatment goals

      b. Discuss possible consequences of surgery; e.g., disfigurement and organ dysfunction resulting from laryngectomy or radical neck dissection

      c. Discuss postsurgical procedures, such as insertion of nasogastric tube and I.V. line and restrictions on oral intake for 10 to 14 days to permit suture line healing

      d. Explain how techniques such as turning, coughing, and deep breathing and early ambulation help prevent postsurgical complications

      e. Perform preoperative bowel preparation, as ordered

      f. Perform aggressive pulmonary hygiene after surgery to prevent pneumonia

      g. Auscultate lungs at least once every shift. Also monitor chest tube drainage and perform necessary tracheostomy care to prevent respiratory complications

      h. Provide chest physiotherapy and encourage turning, coughing, and deep breathing to loosen and expel secretions at least twice a day

     i. Encourage early ambulation to improve respiratory function and reduce the risk of thrombosis

     j. Monitor fluid balance and intervene as necessary to prevent fluid overload

     k. Administer antibiotics, as ordered

     l. Elevate the head of bed to prevent aspiration

    m. Administer analgesics regularly for pain

     n. Give the patient nothing by mouth until suture lines heal and GI tract function returns

     o. Minimize disruption of anastomotic sites by avoiding nasogastric tube manipulation or tension and by maintaining GI decompression with suction

     p. Monitor patency of GI tubes and assess amount and nature of drainage

     q. Notify the physician if a nasogastric tube becomes dislodged; do not attempt to reposition or reinsert it

     r. After the patient's GI function returns, instruct him to remain upright after eating or drinking to prevent reflux or aspiration, and to eat small, frequent meals to prevent gastric distention

     s. Cleanse suture lines according to institutional policy to prevent infection

     t. Take steps to prevent stress on suture lines; e.g., instruct the patient to limit head movement

     u. Teach the patient to avoid maneuvers that can increase intra-abdominal and thoracic pressure (such as Valsalva maneuver and bending at the waist). Explain that such pressure increase can cause reflux and increased stress on suture lines

     v. After laryngectomy, refer the patient to a speech therapist to learn alternate communication methods, such as esophageal speech or use of a mechanical device

    w. Perform meticulous oral hygiene and encourage the patient to brush his teeth and use mouthwash several times a day, and to use mint candies or charcoal carbonate tablets to minimize bad breath

12. Radiotherapeutic interventions

     a. In esophageal cancer, radiation therapy (RT) is used as an adjuvant treatment before and after surgery for cure

     b. RT also may be used to palliate symptoms

     c. Decisions on using RT are based on tumor location

     d. RT may be used alone for upper thoracic esophageal lesions

     e. RT often is used in combination with surgery for lower thoracic esophageal lesions

     f. RT is the primary curative treatment for Stage I and Stage II cervical esophageal lesions

     g. RT represents an alternative to surgery when preservation of the larynx is desired

     h. RT is administered until adverse hematologic and neurologic effects warrant discontinuation or the total maximum dosage is given

        i.   Preoperative purposes of RT include reducing size of tumors that interfere with the patient's ability to eat, thereby improving his nutritional status before surgery; improving tumor resectability; and minimizing tumor dissemination

13. Nursing interventions for patients receiving RT
   a. Provide general nursing care measures applicable to all patients receiving RT (see Section II.C)
   b. Teach the patient and family how to maintain hydration and nutritional status, and stress the importance of doing so even when adverse effects of RT create difficulties
   c. Evaluate the patient's nutritional status weekly, and refer him for nutritional support, if necessary
   d. Encourage the patient with dysphagia or esophagitis to consume liquids and soft foods
   e. Encourage use of nutritional supplements as needed
   f. Provide analgesics, as ordered, to relieve the pain of esophagitis

14. Chemotherapeutic interventions
   a. Chemotherapy is used to increase the effectiveness of RT and to control recurring disease
   b. Chemotherapy has not proven effective in curing esophageal cancer
   c. Agents used include methotrexate, 5-fluorouracil, mitomycin-C, cisplatin, lomustine (CCNU), and doxorubicin
   d. Drugs such as doxorubicin, dactinomycin, and daunorubicin may cause radiation-recall esophagitis and skin reactions

15. Nursing interventions for patients receiving chemotherapy
   a. Provide general nursing care measures applicable to all patients receiving chemotherapy (see Section II.D)
   b. Inform the patient that some agents cause recall esophagitis and skin reactions when used after RT

C. Gastric cancer

1. General information
   a. Most gastric cancers are adenocarcinomas
   b. Lesions may be fungating (rapid-growing), infiltrating, ulcerating, diffuse, or polypoid
   c. Gastric cancer may be well-advanced before clinical manifestations appear

2. Epidemiology
   a. Incidence of gastric cancer is declining
   b. Worldwide, incidence is relatively low in the United States, but highest in Japan where gastric cancer is a leading cause of death
   c. Incidence in blacks is twice that in whites
   d. Peak incidence occurs in men over age 70

3. Risk factors
   a. Environmental exposure to nitrosamines and polycyclic hydrocarbons
   b. Advanced age (risk increases after age 40 and peaks between ages 70 to 80)
   c. Low socioeconomic status
   d. History of poor nutrition
   e. History of achlorhydria gastric polyposis syndrome
   f. History of chronic atrophic gastritis
   g. History of gastric ulcers
   h. History of pernicious anemia
   i. Gastric calcification
4. Clinical manifestations
   a. Vague stomach upset
   b. Vague feeling of abdominal heaviness, especially after meals
   c. Weight loss
   d. Nausea and vomiting
   e. Dysphagia
   f. Anorexia
   g. Palpable or visible abdominal mass
   h. Retrosternal, epigastric, or back pain
   i. Weakness and fatigue
   j. Anemia
   k. Hematemesis
   l. Melena
5. Diagnostic tests
   a. Upper GI series
   b. Gastroscopy
   c. Endoscopic brush biopsy
6. Staging
   a. The TNM system is used to stage gastric cancer
   b. Procedures used in staging include upper GI series, CBC, blood chemistries, chest X-ray, CT scan of chest and abdomen, bone scan (if indicated by blood chemistries), and tumor markers such as serum carcinoembryonic antigen and alpha-fetoprotein
7. Natural progression of disease
   a. Routes of metastasis include lymphatic spread, hematogenous spread, direct extension, and peritoneal seeding
   b. Sites of metastasis include liver, lungs, peritoneum, bone, and ovaries
   c. Prognosis: 5-year survival rate ranges from 60% for Stage I disease to 5% for Stage IV disease
8. Nursing interventions for screening, detection, and prevention
   a. Be aware that no screening or prevention measures exist
   b. Encourage the patient with persistent upper GI tract symptoms to seek prompt medical attention to aid early detection of cancer

9. Nursing interventions for psychosocial needs
   a. Encourage the patient to express feelings about the diagnosis, treatment plan, and impact of the disease on his life-style
   b. Assess patient and family coping mechanisms
   c. Determine the availability of support resources and help the patient gain access to appropriate resources
   d. Promote open communication between the patient and family
   e. Assess the significance of food and eating to the patient (e.g., does eating provide a source of gratification or pleasure, or does it have specific social significance) and evaluate the possible impact of cancer on the patient's ability to eat
10. Surgical interventions
   a. Surgery is the preferred curative treatment modality for gastric cancer
   b. Surgery involves tumor resection, subtotal or total gastrectomy, and regional lymph node dissection
   c. Palliative resection of contiguous organs may be necessary to obtain an adequate margin of tumor-free tissue
   d. Surgical interventions include subtotal esophagogastrectomy, total gastrectomy, or subtotal gastrectomy (Billroth I or Billroth II)
   e. Subtotal gastrectomy (Billroth II) is the preferred procedure when the patient's status permits
11. Nursing interventions for patients undergoing surgery
   a. Provide general nursing care measures applicable to all patients undergoing surgery (see Section II.B)
   b. Discuss with the patient and family probable alterations in GI tract function that will result from surgery
   c. Administer bowel preparation before surgery, as ordered
   d. Monitor patency of drainage tubes, such as nasogastric tubes or wound drains, to maintain gastric decompression
   e. Minimize disruption of anastomotic site by avoiding nasogastric tube manipulation or tension and by maintaining gastric decompression with suction
   f. Notify the physician if the nasogastric tube becomes dislodged; do not attempt to reposition or reinsert it
   g. Monitor the nasogastric tube for signs and symptoms of bleeding or anastomotic leakage
   h. Administer analgesics to relieve pain as necessary
   i. Give the patient nothing by mouth until suture lines heal and GI function returns. Auscultate abdomen for bowel sounds to assess GI function
   j. Monitor gastric pH and intervene as necessary to prevent acid-base imbalance
   k. Teach the patient and family about dietary limitations after surgery; a dietary regimen may involve clear liquids, liquid supplements, low-fat food, or six small meals each day

    l. Assess for signs and symptoms of dumping syndrome, such as pain, severe diarrhea, steatorrhea, and fluid or electrolyte imbalance

    m. As ordered, administer GI anticholinergic agents to slow GI motility and decrease acid secretions

12. Radiotherapeutic interventions

    a. RT effectively palliates symptoms of gastric cancer

    b. Radiation doses of 4,000 to 6,000 rad administered before surgery improves survival rate

    c. RT used in combination with chemotherapy also improves survival rate

13. Nursing interventions for patients receiving RT

    a. Provide general nursing care measures applicable to all patients receiving RT (see Section II.C)

    b. Assess fluid balance and nutritional status and intervene as necessary to prevent dehydration and malnutrition

    c. Observe for nausea, vomiting, and diarrhea and administer medications to control these symptoms as necessary

    d. Monitor serum electrolyte values and intervene as necessary to prevent fluid and electrolyte imbalance

    e. Teach the patient how to maintain optimum nutrition through proper diet and use of nutritional supplements

14. Chemotherapeutic interventions

    a. Chemotherapy has not been established as a standard treatment modality for gastric cancer

    b. Use of chemotherapy as an adjuvant treatment for gastric cancer is under study

    c. Chemotherapy may prolong patient survival in advanced disease

    d. Antineoplastic agents under study include 5-fluorouracil, doxorubicin, mitomycin-C, nitrosoureas, and cisplatin

15. Nursing interventions for patients receiving chemotherapy for gastric cancer involve general nursing care measures applicable to all patients receiving chemotherapy (see Section II.D)

D. Pancreatic cancer

1. General information

    a. Pancreatic cancer typically is widely metastasized at diagnosis

    b. Initial signs and symptoms typically are vague

    c. Surgery represents the only viable curative treatment modality in patients with limited disease

2. Epidemiology

    a. Pancreatic cancer is the seventh most common cancer, accounting for 3% of all cancers

    b. It is the fifth leading cause of cancer death in the United States, accounting for 5% of cancer deaths

    c. Incidence increases with age, peaking at about age 60

    d. Incidence is highest in urban areas

3. Risk factors
   a. Cigarette smoking (doubles risk)
   b. History of alcoholism
   c. History of chronic pancreatitis
   d. History of diabetes mellitus
   e. Chronic exposure to industrial carcinogens such as beta-naphthalene and benzidine
   f. Chronically high dietary fat intake
   g. Advanced age
   h. Urban habitation
   i. Low socioeconomic status
4. Clinical manifestations
   a. Dull pain that gradually increases in intensity
   b. Progressive, obstructive jaundice; present in 80% to 90% of patients
   c. Profound weight loss
   d. Anorexia
   e. Nausea and vomiting
   f. Hemorrhage
   g. Bleeding disorders
   h. Portal hypertension
   i. Hepatomegaly
   j. Gallbladder enlargement
   k. Severe epigastric pain
   l. Splenomegaly
   m. Symptoms of metastatic disease, such as general weakness or sharp upper abdominal pain
   n. Ascites
   o. Sudden onset of diabetes
5. Diagnostic tests
   a. Ultrasonography of pancreas
   b. CT scan of pancreas and abdomen
   c. Magnetic resonance imaging
   d. Endoscopic retrograde cholangiopancreatography (ERCP)
   e. ERCP-directed biopsy or cytology
6. Staging
   a. A variation of the TNM system is being evaluated for use in staging pancreatic cancer
   b. Procedures used in staging include liver function tests, such as SGOT, SGPT, LDH, bilirubin, and alkaline phosphatase levels; chest X-ray; liver scan; bone scan; upper GI series; and selective arteriography, such as celiac angiography
7. Natural progression of disease
   a. Routes of metastasis include local extension, lymphatic spread, hematogenous spread, and peritoneal seeding
   b. Sites of metastasis include regional organs, regional lymph nodes, abdominal cavity, and distant organs

    c. Prognosis: 5-year survival rate is 4%; average survival rate of patients with local extension of disease is 6 months

8. Nursing interventions for screening, detection, and prevention

    a. Keep in mind that no screening procedures for pancreatic cancer exist

    b. Be aware of risk factors and signs and symptoms associated with pancreatic cancer

    c. Refer a patient with possible signs and symptoms of pancreatic cancer for medical evaluation

9. Nursing interventions for psychosocial needs

    a. Encourage the patient to express feelings about the diagnosis, treatment plan, and impact of disease on his life-style

    b. Promote open communication between the patient and family

    c. Anticipate and help meet the patient's and family's needs when prognosis is poor

    d. Reassure the patient that treatment can help manage symptoms

    e. Help family members identify and access appropriate resources as the patient's physical condition deteriorates

    f. Provide emotional support and grief counseling as necessary

10. Surgical interventions

    a. Surgery represents the only possibility for cure of pancreatic cancer

    b. Surgery for pancreatic cancer carries a mortality rate of 15% to 20%

    c. Surgical interventions include total pancreatectomy and pancreatoduodenal resection (Whipple procedure)

    d. Palliative resection may be done to remove tumor, relieve obstructions, or bypass involved organs

    e. The Roux-en-Y procedure, sometimes used for palliative treatment, involves duodenal bypass to relieve obstruction, choledochojejunostomy to relieve icteric pruritus, and celiac ganglion block to control pain

11. Nursing interventions for patients undergoing surgery

    a. Provide general nursing care measures applicable to all patients undergoing surgery (see Section II.B)

    b. Assess for signs and symptoms of infection, abscess formation, and pneumonia

    c. Assess for anastomotic leakage and possible fistula formation

    d. After pancreatectomy, assess for signs and symptoms of diabetes mellitus and monitor blood glucose level for abnormalities

    e. Assess for signs and symptoms of peptic ulceration

    f. Give the patient nothing by mouth until GI function returns

    g. Evaluate nutritional status; assess ability to eat and absorb nutrients, such as protein and fats, when GI function returns

    h. Evaluate for malabsorption of fat and protein resulting from loss of pancreatic tissue

    i. Provide small, frequent meals to prevent effects similar to those of dumping syndrome

    j. Encourage the patient to avoid caffeine and alcohol to prevent excessive
       gastric acidity
    k. Teach the patient and family about enzyme replacement therapy and the
       patient's special dietary needs
    l. As ordered, administer replacement pancreatic enzymes such as lipase,
       amylase, and trypsin to reduce steatorrhea
    m. As ordered, administer gastric acid inhibitors to reduce steatorrhea and
       diarrhea and to slow weight loss
    n. As appropriate, teach the patient and family measures to control diabetes
       mellitus, including diet and exercise guidelines, insulin administration,
       and blood glucose monitoring
12. Radiotherapeutic interventions
    a. RT has not proven effective as a primary treatment modality in
       pancreatic cancer
    b. External beam therapy, interstitial implants, and intraoperative RT do not
       significantly effect survival rate
    c. RT's ineffectiveness in treating pancreatic cancer is largely attributed to
       the typically advanced disease stage at diagnosis
    d. Combined use of chemotherapy and RT palliates pain in about half of
       patients treated and increases survival time in some patients
13. Nursing interventions for patients receiving RT
    a. Provide general nursing care measures applicable to all patients receiving
       RT (see Section II.C)
    b. Inform the patient and family that the patient may develop diabetes
       mellitus as a result of therapy. Discuss glucose monitoring and insulin
       administration, as appropriate
14. Chemotherapeutic interventions
    a. Single-agent and combination chemotherapy do not improve survival rate
       in pancreatic cancer
    b. Chemotherapy may be used for symptom palliation
    c. Survival rate improves slightly when chemotherapy is used as a
       radiosensitizer for RT
    d. Agents used include 5-fluorouracil, mitomycin-C, streptozotocin,
       doxorubicin, and methotrexate
15. Nursing interventions for patients receiving chemotherapy for pancreatic
    cancer involve general nursing care measures applicable to all patients
    receiving chemotherapy (see Section II.D)

E. Liver cancer

1. General information
   a. Primary liver cancers are adenocarcinomas, classified by cell type as
      hepatocellular carcinomas (arising from parenchymal cells), accounting
      for 70% to 90% of all liver cancers; cholangiocarcinomas (arising from
      hepatic bile ducts), representing 10% to 30% of all liver cancers; and
      mixed cellular forms, which rarely occur

      b. Major complications include esophageal varices and ascites; hemorrhage from obstruction, necrosis, or rupture of the portal vein can be fatal

      c. Liver failure is the primary cause of death associated with liver cancer

2. Epidemiology

      a. Liver cancer accounts for less than 2% of all cancers diagnosed in the United States

      b. Incidence in men is six to ten times greater than in women

      c. Onset typically occurs between ages 60 and 70

3. Risk factors

      a. Cirrhosis of liver caused by alcoholism, hepatitis, hemachromatosis, or alpha-antitrypsin deficiency

      b. History of hepatitis B infection

      c. Prolonged malnutrition

      d. Consumption of food contaminated with aflatoxin, such as aspergillus flavus

      e. Exposure to thorotrast (once used as a contrast medium), polyvinyl chloride, and nitrosamines

      f. Infestation with liver flukes or parasites

4. Clinical manifestations

      a. Dull, aching pain in the abdominal right upper quadrant (RUQ)

      b. Palpable mass in the RUQ

      c. Liver tenderness

      d. Profound, progressive weakness

      e. Feelings of epigastric fullness

      f. Constipation or diarrhea

      g. Anorexia

      h. Weight loss

      i. Ascites

      j. Jaundice

      k. Cholecystitis

      l. Recurrent hepatitis

      m. Sudden onset of portal hypertension

5. Diagnostic tests

      a. Liver biopsy

      b. Liver function tests, such as SGOT, SGPT, LDH, and alkaline phosphatase

      c. Alpha-fetoprotein levels

6. Staging

      a. No definitive staging system for liver cancer exists

      b. Procedures used in staging include chest X-ray, abdominal ultrasonography, liver scan, abdominal CT scan, and angiography of the spleen, liver, and inferior vena cava

7. Natural progression of disease

      a. Routes of metastasis include direct extension (most common), lymphatic spread, and hematogenous spread

      b. Sites of metastasis include regional lymph nodes, lungs, and brain

    c. Prognosis: 5-year survival rate is less than 2%; patients with inoperable liver cancer typically survive less than 6 months

8. Nursing interventions for screening, detection, and prevention
    a. Keep in mind that no screening procedures for liver cancer exist
    b. Be aware of the risk factors and clinical manifestations associated with liver cancer
    c. Refer a patient displaying possible signs and symptoms of liver cancer for medical evaluation

9. Nursing interventions for psychosocial needs
    a. Encourage the patient to express feelings about the diagnosis, treatment plan, and impact of disease on his life-style
    b. Assess patient and family coping mechanisms
    c. Promote open communication between the patient and family
    d. Anticipate and help meet the patient's and family's needs when prognosis is poor
    e. Explain that treatment may help manage symptoms
    f. Help the patient and family identify and access appropriate resources as the patient's physical condition deteriorates
    g. Provide emotional support and grief counseling as necessary

10. Surgical interventions
    a. Wide en bloc tumor excision is the preferred curative treatment for solitary, localized lesions
    b. Surgery usually is ineffective and contraindicated in extensive or advanced disease
    c. Selective surgery may provide symptom palliation
    d. The presence of cirrhosis increases the surgical risk
    e. Liver transplant in certain circumstances is under investigation

11. Nursing interventions for patients undergoing surgery
    a. Provide general nursing care measures applicable to all patients undergoing surgery (see Section II.B)
    b. Assess for clotting defects; findings may include delayed prothrombin time, hematuria, or CBC abnormalities
    c. Administer vitamin K as needed to prevent hemorrhage
    d. Assess for pneumonia and atelectasis; auscultate lung bases for fluid, which may indicate subphrenic abscess
    e. Perform aggressive pulmonary hygiene, including turning, coughing, and deep breathing every 2 hours during waking hours to prevent respiratory complications
    f. Care for wound and drainage tube sites according to institutional protocol to prevent infection
    g. Assess abdominal girth to detect bleeding or monitor progression of ascites
    h. Evaluate laboratory test results for signs of liver dysfunction, such as elevated liver enzymes, SGOT, or bilirubin levels

      i.   Intervene as necessary to help control pruritus associated with jaundice; for instance, provide meticulous skin care, apply topical lotions, and administer oral antihistamines or cholestyramine as ordered

      j.   Maintain patency and position of drainage tubes

      k.   Assess T-tube for proper placement and for amount and nature of drainage; drainage exceeding 400 ml per day indicates fistula

      l.   Check central venous pressure for signs of portal hypertension

      m. Be alert for RUQ pain and low-grade fever, which may indicate subphrenic abscess

12. Radiotherapeutic interventions

      a.   Applications of RT in liver cancer are limited to palliative treatment

      b.   The liver's radiation tolerance remains uncertain

      c.   Concomitant use of RT and chemotherapy is under investigation

13. Nursing implications for patients receiving RT

      a.   Provide general nursing care measures applicable to all patients receiving RT (see Section II.C)

      b.   Assess for nausea and vomiting and intervene as necessary to control these symptoms

14. Chemotherapeutic interventions

      a.   Chemotherapy is the preferred treatment modality for unresectable liver cancer

      b.   It also is used as an adjuvant treatment after surgery

      c.   Combination chemotherapy has produced the best results; single-agent chemotherapy is less effective

      d.   Use of chemotherapy in combination with RT is under investigation

      e.   Antineoplastic agents once were routinely infused into the portal vein to minimize systemic toxicity. Now, however, the hepatic artery—the primary blood supply for liver tumors—is the preferred infusion site

      f.   Hepatic artery infusion delivers high drug concentrations to the liver and minimizes systemic toxicity

      g.   Hepatic artery infusion requires insertion of a catheter into the hepatic artery to deliver continuous drug infusion, regulated by an external or implanted infusion pump

15. Nursing interventions for patients receiving chemotherapy

      a.   Provide general nursing care measures applicable to all patients receiving chemotherapy (see Section II.D)

      b.   Discuss the treatment plan with the patient and family, including rationale for administering chemotherapy as an infusion into the portal vein or hepatic artery

F. Colorectal cancer

1. General information

      a.   Colorectal cancer typically develops slowly

      b.   Symptoms usually appear early, but metastasis occurs late

    c. Adenocarcinomas account for 95% to 98% of all colon cancers

    d. Location of colorectal cancer depends on histologic cell type. Squamous cell cancers form at the anal verge; basal cell cancers, at the anal verge and in the perianal area; and malignant melanomas, in the perianal area; lymphomas and sarcomas rarely occur

    e. Rectal cancers recur more often than colonic tumors

    f. Most colorectal cancers develop from a benign adenomatous polyp

    g. Prophylactic removal of polyps reduces the incidence of colorectal cancer

2. Epidemiology

    a. Each year in the United States, approximately 147,000 cases of colorectal cancer are diagnosed

    b. Colorectal cancer is the second most common cancer in women, the third most common in men

    c. It is the third leading cause of cancer death in women, the second leading cause in men

    d. Colorectal cancer may occur at any age; incidence increases starting at age 40

    e. Average age at diagnosis is 60

    f. Men and women are at equal risk

    g. Lower-than-average incidence has been recorded in members of religious sects that restrict meat consumption

    h. Patients with a family history of colon cancer usually develop the disease at a younger age than patients with no family history of colon cancer

3. Risk factors

    a. Excessive dietary fat intake (increases risk)

    b. Excessive bile acids in the GI tract

    c. Low dietary fiber intake

    d. History of sporadic colonic polyps and polyposis syndromes

    e. History of familial polyposis coli (most untreated patients develop colorectal cancer)

    f. Family history of colon cancer (triples risk)

    g. History of ulcerative colitis (considered a premalignant condition)

    h. History of Crohn's disease

    i. Chronic exposure to carcinogens, such as asbestos, nitrosamines, and tryptophan metabolites

4. Clinical manifestations

    a. Vary according to tumor location; manifestations common to all locations include blood in stool; vague, dull pain; obstruction; and a change in bowel habits

    b. Ascending colon (appear after tumors become large and bulky): palpable mass, anemia, occult bleeding, acute pain and shock resulting from perforation, and obstruction (rare because of lumen size and liquid quality of stool)

    c. Transverse colon: change in bowel habits, blood in stool, and obstruction

    d. Descending and sigmoid colon: vague abdominal pain, gas pain, constipation, reduced caliber of stool, blood in stool, and obstruction

     e. Rectum: bright red blood in stool, sensation of incomplete evacuation, tenesmus, and mucous diarrhea

5. Diagnostic tests
    a. Digital rectal examination
    b. Fecal occult blood screening
    c. Proctosigmoidoscopy
    d. Barium enema
    e. Colonoscopy
    f. Endoscopy-directed biopsy

6. Staging
    a. The Aster-Coller modification of Duke's classification system usually is used to stage colorectal cancer. The TNM system also may be used
    b. Procedures used in staging include blood chemistries, especially liver function tests such as SGOT and bilirubin levels; serum carcinoembryonic antigen levels; chest X-ray; liver scan (if indicated by blood chemistries or hepatomegaly); bone scan (if indicated by blood chemistries); CT scan of the abdomen and pelvis

7. Natural progression of disease
    a. Routes of metastasis include bowel wall penetration; lymphatic and vascular channel invasion after penetration of submucosal layer of bowel; and local structure invasion (more common in cecum and rectosigmoid area)
    b. Sites of metastasis include liver (most common site), lungs (common site), adrenal glands, ovaries, bone, and peritoneum
    c. Prognosis: 5-year survival rate ranges from 75% to 100% for Stage A disease to 5% for Stage D disease

8. Nursing interventions for screening, detection, and prevention
    a. Teach patients about dietary risk factors
    b. Encourage them to make appropriate dietary changes, such as reducing dietary fat and increasing dietary fiber intake
    c. Screen stool for occult blood
    d. Encourage high-risk patients to have regular check-ups (at least once a year), including digital rectal examinations
    e. Encourage all patients age 40 or older to have annual digital rectal examinations
    f. Teach patients about preventive surgical procedures to treat premalignant lesions

9. Nursing interventions for psychosocial needs
    a. Encourage the patient to express feelings about the diagnosis, treatment plan, and impact of disease on his life-style
    b. Assess patient and family coping mechanisms
    c. Determine the availability of support resources and help the patient gain access to such appropriate resources
    d. Evaluate the patient's reaction to planned procedures, such as colostomy formation, which may alter his body image

e. Discuss the possible effects of cancer and colostomy on the patient's sexual function and identity

10. Surgical interventions
    a. Surgery is used for prophylaxis, cure, or palliation
    b. Prophylactic surgery prevents certain high-risk GI disorders, such as diverticulitis and polyps, from developing into malignancies
    c. Prophylactic surgeries include polypectomy, total colectomy, ileostomy, and proctocolectomy
    d. Primary resection is the preferred curative treatment
    e. Primary resection procedures include resection with primary anastomosis, resection with temporary colostomy (two-stage procedure), and resection with permanent colostomy
    f. Abdominal-perineal (A-P) resection is used for lower rectal tumors
    g. Palliative surgery may provide pain relief, or prevent or relieve bowel obstruction

11. Nursing interventions for patients undergoing surgery
    a. Provide general nursing care measures applicable to all patients undergoing surgery (see Section II.B)
    b. Assist with preoperative bowel preparation, as ordered
    c. As appropriate, refer the patient to an enterostomal therapist before surgery for colostomy site selection and marking
    d. Assess for signs and symptoms of postoperative urinary tract injury or infection
    e. Assess for return of bowel function by auscultating for bowel sounds and assess for signs and symptoms of paralytic ileus
    f. Give the patient nothing by mouth until GI function returns
    g. Assess colostomy circulation and function; evaluate stoma for color and appearance (for example, prolapse or retraction)
    h. Assess perineal wound healing in A-P resections
    i. Regularly check patency and function of GI tubes, suction machines, drains, and catheters
    j. Provide wound, drain site, perineal, and peristomal skin care
    k. Teach the patient and family proper colostomy care procedures
    l. Explain the normal consistency and frequency of colostomy output, depending on the area and extent of bowel resection and the type of colostomy formed. For instance, frequent loose stools should be expected from an ascending colostomy; daily firm stools, from a sigmoid colostomy
    m. Explain the importance of adequate hydration for bowel evacuation
    n. Institute dietary modifications to control colostomy odor and gas
    o. Teach proper irrigation techniques to the patient with a sigmoid or descending colostomy
    p. Encourage the patient to change appliances as needed
    q. Refer the patient to ostomy organizations and other support groups as necessary

12. Radiotherapeutic interventions
    a. RT has limited applications in treating colon cancer; use is mainly palliative
    b. RT is a primary curative therapy for rectal cancer in patients not considered candidates for surgery
    c. It also may be used before surgery for rectal cancer to reduce tumor size and facilitate resection, and after surgery for rectal cancer to inhibit local recurrence
    d. It also may be used to palliate pain and complications of metastasis in rectal cancer
13. Nursing interventions for patients receiving RT
    a. Provide general nursing care measures applicable to all patients receiving RT (see Section II.C)
    b. Assess for changes in condition of irradiated skin; keep in mind that enterocutaneous fistula may result from RT
    c. Assess elimination patterns; observe for diarrhea resulting from irradiation to the abdomen
    d. Maintain adequate fluid intake and intervene as necessary to prevent dehydration and fluid and electrolyte imbalance
    e. Evaluate the effects of changes in elimination on colostomy and peristomal skin; provide meticulous skin care, and teach the patient how to keep peristomal skin clean, dry, and intact
    f. Modify diet as necessary to minimize nausea, vomiting, and diarrhea
14. Chemotherapeutic interventions
    a. Use of chemotherapy alone does not improve survival rate in patients with colorectal cancer
    b. Chemotherapy is used predominantly following surgery in patients with advanced disease
    c. Antineoplastic agents used include 5-fluorouracil, lomustine, cisplatin, vincristine, and methotrexate
    d. Antineoplastic agents may be administered through hepatic artery infusion to treat patients with liver metastasis
    e. Floxuridine (FUDR) is the drug most often used in hepatic artery infusion
15. Nursing interventions for patients receiving chemotherapy
    a. Provide general nursing care measures applicable to all patients receiving chemotherapy (see Section II.D)
    b. Assess liver function tests before starting hepatic artery infusion
    c. If anticoagulants are given to prevent catheter-induced thrombosis, assess coagulation studies for abnormalities
    d. As appropriate, teach the patient and family precautions for anticoagulant use
    e. Teach the patient and family how to use and care for hepatic artery infusion equipment

Points to Remember

GI tract cancer typically has an insidious onset and often is metastasized by the time of diagnosis.

Surgery is the preferred treatment for localized GI tract cancers.

Primary risk factors for gastric cancer are environmental in nature.

Blood in the stool is an important sign of possible colorectal cancer.

Clinical manifestations and treatment of esophageal and colorectal cancer vary according to tumor location.

A patient with GI tract cancer requires careful nutritional assessment and effective interventions to maintain nutritional status.

A patient requiring a colostomy as part of his treatment for colon cancer requires comprehensive nursing interventions to aid his adaptation to the colostomy.

Glossary

Achalasia—esophageal obstruction proximal to the cardioesophageal junction

Achlorhydria—absence of hydrochloric acid in gastric juices

Ascites—abnormal fluid accumulation in the peritoneal cavity

Jaundice—yellowing of skin and eyes caused by excessive bile pigment in the blood

Steatorrhea—presence of excessive fat in stool resulting from malabsorption of fat; caused by disease of intestinal mucosa or pancreatic enzyme deficiency

Tylosis—syndrome characterized by hyperkeratosis of the palms or soles; a risk factor associated with esophageal cancer

Cancer of the Urinary Tract

Learning Objectives
After studying this section, the reader should be able to:

• Discuss the epidemiology and risk factors for urinary tract cancers.

• List possible clinical manifestations of each cancer.

• Identify several tests used to diagnose and stage each cancer.

• Discuss common routes of dissemination for each cancer.

• Identify several medical and surgical interventions for each cancer.

• Discuss nursing interventions for patients undergoing treatment for urinary tract cancer.

X. Cancer of the Urinary Tract

A. Introduction
1. Renal and bladder cancers are common in adult men and women
2. Two types of renal cancer exist
   a. Renal cell carcinoma
   b. Cancer of the renal pelvis
3. Cigarette smoking is a important risk factor for both renal and bladder cancers

B. Renal cancer
1. General information
   a. The etiology of renal cancer remains unclear
   b. Renal cell carcinomas form in tubular epithelial cells of the parenchyma
   c. Cancer of the renal pelvis develop from transitional cells or squamous cells, and may occur anywhere in the renal pelvis
2. Epidemiology
   a. Renal cancer represents approximately 3% of all cancers diagnosed in the United States
   b. Renal cell carcinomas—also known as hypernephroma and renal adenocarcinomas—account for 85% of renal cancers. Cancer of the renal pelvis accounts for 5% to 9% of renal cancers
   c. Incidence is twice as high in men than in women
   d. Incidence is higher in Scandinavian countries and lower in Japan; incidence in the United States is about equal to worldwide average
   e. Incidence increases with age
   f. Occurrence is rare in patients under age 35; age at diagnosis usually ranges from 55 to 60
3. Risk factors
   a. Cigarette smoking
   b. Urban habitition
   c. Family history of renal cell cancer
   d. Exposure to thorotrast (once used as a contrast medium)
   e. Phenacetin use (increases risk of renal pelvis cancer)
4. Clinical manifestations
   a. Gross hematuria (a classic sign and the presenting complaint in 40% of patients)
   b. Dull flank pain (classic symptom)
   c. Palpable abdominal mass (classic sign)
   d. Fever
   e. Weight loss
   f. Anemia
   g. Hypercalcemia
5. Diagnostic tests
   a. Urinalysis
   b. X-ray of kidneys, ureters, and bladder (KUB)
   c. Intravenous pyelography (IVP)

    d. Renal angiography
    e. Urinary cytology
    f. Nephrotomography
    g. Renal ultrasonography
6. Staging
    a. A modified Flocks and Kadesky staging system, or possibly the tumor, node, metastasis (TNM) system, is used to stage renal cell carcinoma
    b. No official staging system exists for cancer of the renal pelvis
    c. Procedures used in staging include blood chemistries to examine renal, bone, and liver function, chest X-ray, liver scan (if liver metastasis is suspected), bone scan (if bone metastasis is suspected), and computed tomography (CT) scan of the brain (if signs of neurologic involvement develop)
7. Natural progression of disease
    a. Routes of metastasis for both types of renal cancer include direct extension, lymphatic spread, and hematogenous spread
    b. Sites of metastasis for both types of renal cancer include ipsilateral renal hilus, regional and distant lymph nodes, vena cava, perinephric fat, lungs, liver, and bone
    c. Prognosis for both types: 30% to 50% of patients have metastatic disease when diagnosed; 5-year survival rate ranges from 65% to 70% for Stage I disease to less than 10% for Stage IV disease
8. Nursing interventions for screening, detection, and prevention
    a. Remember that no screening tests for renal cancer exist
    b. Teach patients to eliminate or minimize exposure to risk factors, such as cigarette smoking
    c. Help a patient arrange prompt medical treatment if signs and symptoms develop
9. Nursing interventions for psychosocial needs
    a. Encourage the patient to express feelings regarding diagnosis, treatment plan, and impact of disease on his life-style
    b. Assess patient and family coping mechanisms
    c. Determine the availability of support resources and help the patient gain access to appropriate resources
    d. Assess the patient's anxiety regarding possible loss of renal function and dependency on dialysis
    e. Assure the patient that one functioning kidney can sustain life
10. Surgical interventions
    a. Radical nephrectomy is the preferred treatment for renal cell carcinoma
    b. Partial nephrectomy is used if only one kidney is functioning; may be used in bilateral renal disease
    c. Between 1 and 7 days before nephrectomy for renal cell carcinoma, the renal vein or artery must be occluded to prevent tumor embolization during surgical manipulation. This reduces tumor vascularity and amplifies the body's immunologic response to the tumor

    d. Preferred surgery for cancer of the renal pelvis involves resection of the affected kidney, surrounding tissue, lymph nodes, ureter, and the periureteral section of the bladder

    e. Surgery also is used as an adjunctive treatment in metastic disease to enhance immunologic response and improve survival rate

    f. Surgery also may be used to palliate symptoms, such as pain

11. Nursing interventions for patients undergoing surgery

    a. Provide general nursing care measures applicable to all patients undergoing surgery (see section II.B)

    b. As appropriate, discuss the rationale for surgically induced renal vein or artery infarction and explain possible complications of this procedure

    c. As ordered, administer medications for pain, fever, and nausea related to renal vein or artery infarction

    d. Assess for postoperative hemorrhage; keep in mind that the kidney is a highly vascular organ prone to hemorrhage

    e. Assess respiratory function for possible pneumothorax after radical nephrectomy is done using the thoracoabdominal approach

    f. Assess fluid and electrolyte balance, and monitor laboratory test results for abnormalities

    g. Assess function of remaining kidney

12. Radiotherapeutic interventions

    a. Because most renal tumors are radioresistant, radiation therapy (RT) is of little value in treatment

    b. RT may be used to palliate bleeding, pain, or symptoms of metastatic disease

    c. Some authorities advocate using RT in conjunction with surgery to reduce the incidence of local recurrence

13. Nursing interventions for patients receiving RT for renal cancer consist of those general nursing care measures applicable to all patients receiving RT (see section II.C)

14. Chemotherapeutic interventions

    a. Chemotherapy occasionally has been used to treat cancer of the renal pelvis, but with little success

    b. Metastatic renal cell carcinoma also does not respond well to cytotoxic chemotherapy

    c. Vinblastine (Velban) has achieved some response in treating renal cell carcinoma

    d. Hormonal agents, including medroxyprogesterone acetate and megestrol acetate, have a minimal effect on renal cell carcinoma

    e. Response to immunotherapy using Bacillus Calmette-Guérin, immune RNA, transfer factor, and autologous tumor cells has been transient and insignificant

    f. Interferon has achieved limited response

15. Nursing interventions for patients receiving chemotherapy for renal cancer consists of general nursing care measures applicable to all patients receiving chemotherapy (see section II.D)

C. Bladder cancer
1. General information
   a. Bladder cancer is usually a multifocal disease of the urinary tract lining (urothelium)
   b. It typically develops on the bladder floor and occasionally involves ureteral orifices
   c. Clinical manifestations of bladder cancer often mimic those of benign prostatic hypertrophy, possibly interfering with diagnosis
   d. Transitional cell carcinomas account for 90% to 95% of all bladder cancers: squamous cell carcinomas, 5% to 10%; and adenocarcinomas, 2% to 3%
   e. Tumors may be papillary (nipple-shaped), carcinoma in situ (CIS), or solid
   f. Papillary tumors are usually low-grade, noninvasive tumors that have a high incidence of recurrence
   g. Transitional CIS typically involves multiple centers of tumor growth
2. Epidemiology
   a. Bladder cancers represent 4% to 5% of all cancers diagnosed in the United States
   b. Incidence is three times higher in men than in women
   c. Peak incidence occurs after age 50
   d. Incidence in white men is twice that in black and Hispanic men
   e. Worldwide, the highest incidence occurs in Africa and the Middle East
3. Risk factors
   a. Cigarette smoking
   b. Chronic exposure to industrial agents such as aniline dye, beta-naphthalene, benzidine, and aminobiphenyl
   c. Chronic ingestion of chemicals such as phenacetin, caffeine, sodium saccharin, sodium cyclamate, or cyclophosphamide
   d. History of bladder infection from *Schistosoma haematobium* (associated with squamous cell bladder cancer), a condition endemic in regions of Africa and the Middle East
   e. History of pelvic irradiation
   f. Abnormal tryptophan metabolism
4. Clinical manifestations
   a. Gross, painless hematuria
   b. Dysuria
   c. Urinary urgency
   d. Urinary frequency
   e. Burning on urination
   f. Urinary hesitancy
   g. Pelvic discomfort after voiding
   h. Decrease in caliber or force of the urine stream
   i. Flank pain
   j. Hydroureter
   k. Hydronephrosis

5. Diagnostic tests
   a. Urinalysis
   b. Cystoscopy
   c. Urine cytology
   d. Endoscopic biopsy
6. Staging
   a. Both the modified Jewett-Strong and the TNM systems are used for staging bladder cancer
   b. Procedures used in staging include blood chemistries, chest X-ray, IVP, liver scan (if indicated by blood chemistries), bone scan (if indicated by blood chemistries), CT scan of abdomen and pelvis (focusing on lymph nodes), and lymphangiography (if nodal involvement is suspected)
7. Natural progression of disease
   a. Routes of metastasis include direct extension, growth through muscle wall and serosal lining into adjacent structures, lymphatic spread, and hematogenous spread
   b. Sites of metastasis include adjacent structures, bone, liver, and lungs
   c. Prognosis depends on depth of tumor penetration into bladder wall, with transitional cell carcinomas carrying the best prognosis; 5-year survival rate for patients with bladder cancer ranges from 80% for Stage 0 and Stage A disease to less than 10% for Stage D disease
8. Nursing interventions for screening, detection, and prevention
   a. Keep in mind that no screening tests for bladder cancer exist
   b. Inform patients of risk factors for bladder cancer
   c. Help arrange prompt medical attention for a patient with possible signs and symptoms of bladder cancer
9. Nursing interventions for psychosocial needs
   a. Encourage the patient to express feelings regarding diagnosis, treatment plan, and impact of disease on his life-style
   b. Assess patient and family coping mechanisms
   c. Determine the availability of support resources and help the patient gain access to appropriate resources
   d. Discuss expected changes in the patient's body image following treatment, such as urinary diversion
   e. Encourage the patient to discuss how cancer and the urinary diversion will affect his sexual function and identity
   f. Inform the patient that radical surgery may cause impotence; encourage him to express feelings, and provide emotional support
   g. Provide appropriate patient teaching for a patient scheduled to receive a penile implant
   h. Provide emotional support for the patient and his partner before and after insertion of a penile implant
10. Surgical interventions
    a. Transurethral resection (TUR) or fulguration is the treatment of choice for superficial low-grade tumors and CIS

      b. Partial or segmental cystectomy is used for tumors on the bladder dome, solitary lesions, and when a tumor-free margin of 3 cm (1¼″) or more is available; recurrence is common after these procedures, however

      c. Radical cystectomy (prostatocystectomy) is used for diffuse, multifocal, recurring, and superficial high-grade tumors; severe CIS; and invasive tumors. RT may be administered before surgery

      d. In men, radical cystectomy involves resection of the bladder, urethra, perivesical fat, attached peritoneum, prostate gland, and seminal vesicle; impotence results from nerve disruption

      e. In women, radical cystectomy involves resection of the bladder, urethra, uterus, ovaries, fallopian tubes, and anterior vaginal wall

      f. Bladder resection necessitates creation of a urinary diversion, such as ileal conduit, bowel conduit, loop stoma, ureterosigmoidostomy, or continent ileal reservoir

11. Nursing interventions for patients undergoing surgery

      a. Provide general nursing care measures applicable to all patients undergoing surgery (see Section II.B)

      b. Assist with preoperative bowel preparation as needed

      c. Refer the patient to an enterostomal therapist before surgery for ostomy site selection and marking

      d. After surgery, assess the urethral meatus for signs of bleeding and the surgical site for complications

      e. Maintain patency of urinary catheter and irrigation tubes to prevent fluid accumulation and bladder spasms

      f. Maintain continuous bladder irrigation to dislodge blood clots following TUR

      g. Monitor intake and output and intervene as necessary to maintain fluid balance

      h. Assess color of urine; may be pale red at first, becoming pale pink. Notify physician of bright red urine, which indicates hemorrhage

      i. Assess for signs and symptoms of fluid overload, infection, obstruction, and hemorrhage

      j. Inform the patient that because partial or segmental cystectomy reduces bladder capacity, he will need to urinate more often

      k. Teach the patient and family about radical cystectomy, including the need for urinary diversion and the likelihood of impotence following surgery (for men)

      l. Observe the urinary diversion site for immediate urine flow

      m. Assess the function and integrity of the urinary diversion

      n. Assess placement of ureteral stents in the ostomy bag, done to prevent formation of ureteral strictures at anastomotic sites

      o. Ensure proper positioning of urinary appliance to maintain integrity of peristomal skin and incision line

      p. Observe stoma color (should be pink to red) to assess circulation; notify physician if stoma becomes dusky or appears necrotic

q. Ensure continuous urine drainage by removing any blood or mucous plugs from ostomy site (some mucous is normal when the bowel is used as a conduit)

r. Instruct the patient to increase fluid intake to at least 3000 ml per day

s. Teach the patient and family proper ostomy care and pouch application; explain that the appliance opening should be adjusted as the stoma shrinks over time

t. Refer the patient to a visiting nursing service for home care follow-up, if necessary

u. Stress the importance of regular medical follow-up examinations

v. Refer the patient and family to ostomy organizations for support

12. Radiotherapeutic interventions

a. In bladder cancer, RT is used before surgery for high-grade, invasive lesions; after segmental resection of high-grade tumors; and alone to palliate pain secondary to bone metastasis and hemorrhage

b. RT applied before radical cystectomy is the optimal treatment for high-grade, high-stage tumors

c. Although using RT before surgery is not associated with increased survival rate, it does seem to reduce the rate of local recurrence

d. RT used as an adjuvant to chemotherapy is under investigation

13. Nursing interventions for patients receiving RT for bladder cancer consist of those general nursing care measures applicable to all patients receiving RT (see Section II.C)

14. Chemotherapeutic interventions

a. Topical (intravesical) chemotherapy is preferred for superficial, low-grade bladder cancers; it is not effective in CIS, however

b. Intravesical chemotherapy reduces the rate of cancer recurrence

c. Intravesical chemotherapy is administered in the operating room or nursing unit after TUR

d. The diluted drug is instilled in an empty bladder and left for 1 to 2 hours or as ordered; number of repetitions depends on the drug used

e. Commonly used agents include thiotepa (most often), mitomycin-C, bleomycin, and cisplatin

f. Systemic chemotherapy using single agents or combinations has proved somewhat effective, but response is temporary

g. Commonly used agents include cyclophosphamide, doxorubicin, cisplatin, and 5-fluorouracil

15. Nursing interventions for patients receiving chemotherapy

a. Provide general nursing care measures applicable to all patients receiving chemotherapy (see Section II.D)

b. Assess the patient for adverse effects, such as severe bladder irritation or myelosuppression

c. Stress the importance of comprehensive follow-up examinations; cystoscopic examination, urine cytologies, and biopsies of suspicious tissues are usually performed every 3 months

Points to Remember

The three classic signs and symptoms of renal cancer are gross hematuria, dull flank pain, and a palpable abdominal mass.

Prognosis for patients with renal cell cancer is unfavorable.

Surgically induced renal vein or artery infarction performed before surgical resection amplifies the body's immunologic response to the tumor.

Clinical manifestations of bladder cancer may mimic symptoms of benign prostatic hypertrophy, possibly interfering with diagnosis.

Transurethral resection or fulguration, alone or in conjunction with intravesical chemotherapy, often controls early-stage bladder cancer.

Cystectomy necessitates creation of a urinary diversion.

Nursing care for a patient with a urinary diversion focuses on helping the patient cope with altered body function and self-image.

Glossary

Segmental cystectomy—surgical procedure involving partial bladder removal

Transurethral fulguration—electrosurgical procedure involving insertion of an instrument into the urethra and destruction of tissue with electrical current

Urothelium—epithelial lining of the urinary tract

Cancer of the Reproductive Tract

Learning Objectives

After studying this section, the reader should be able to:

- Discuss the epidemiology and risk factors for each major type of reproductive tract cancer.

- List possible clinical manifestations of each cancer.

- Identify several tests used to diagnose and stage each cancer.

- Discuss common routes of dissemination for each cancer.

- Identify several medical and surgical interventions for each cancer.

- Describe nursing interventions for patients undergoing treatment for reproductive tract cancer.

XI. Cancer of the Reproductive Tract

A. **Introduction**
  1. Reproductive tract cancer typically poses a serious threat to a patient's physiologic and psychological status
  2. Patients with reproductive tract cancer often face difficult psychosexual adjustments resulting from:
     a. Tumor location
     b. Threat to body image posed by tumor removal
     c. Effects of disease and treatment on sexual function and identity
  3. The type of tumor cell directs choice of treatment modality
  4. Types of cancer cells involved in reproductive tract cancer are as follows:
     a. Squamous cell carcinomas are prevalent in the cervix
     b. Adenocarcinomas typically develop in the prostate gland and ovaries
     c. Germ cell tumors typically develop in the testes
  5. Early detection of cervical cancer using the Papanicolaou (Pap) test has reduced the mortality rate associated with cervical cancer

B. **Prostatic cancer**
  1. General information
     a. The cause of prostatic cancer remains unknown
     b. Adenocarcinoma is the prevalent form of prostatic cancer
     c. The typical clinical presentation is an elderly man experiencing weight loss, back pain, and prostatism
     d. Prostatic cancer often is asymptomatic in early stages, or may manifest signs and symptoms mimicking those of benign prostatic hypertrophy
     e. Sudden onset and rapid progression of symptoms may indicate prostatic cancer
     f. Observation is a treatment option for early-stage, low-grade lesions
  2. Epidemiology
     a. Prostatic cancer accounts for approximately 20% of all cancers in men in the United States
     b. Prostatic cancer accounts for approximately 11% of cancer deaths in men in the United States
     c. American blacks have the highest incidence of prostatic cancer in the world
     d. Incidence in all men rises after age 40 and peaks between ages 60 and 70
  3. Risk factors
     a. Chronic occupational exposure to cadmium, zinc, or rubber
     b. Increased testosterone levels (possibly)
  4. Clinical manifestations
     a. Urinary hesitancy
     b. Urinary frequency
     c. Urinary urgency

      d. Decreased caliber and force of urine stream
      e. Urinary dribbling
      f. Hematuria
      g. Back pain
      h. Pelvic pain
      i. Urinary incontinence
5. Diagnostic tests
      a. Rectal examination
      b. Transrectal or transperineal needle biopsy
      c. Evaluation of prostatic fluid
      d. Serum prostatic acid phosphatase testing
      e. Urine cytology
6. Staging
      a. Prostatic caner is staged using the tumor, node, metastasis (TNM) system or another staging system based on clinical estimates of tumor involvement
      b. Procedures used in staging include complete blood count (CBC), blood chemistries, urinalysis, chest X-ray, intravenous pyelography (IVP), bone scan, computer tomography (CT) scan of pelvis, lymphangiography, and lactic dehydrogenase isoenzyme testing
7. Natural progression of disease
      a. Routes of metastasis include local extension to surrounding structures, lymphatic spread, and hematogenous spread
      b. Sites of metastasis include lymph nodes, vertebrae, pelvis, femur, rib, lungs, liver, and kidneys
      c. Prognosis varies greatly with tumor grade and stage of disease; 10-year survival rate ranges from 60% for Stage A disease to 10% for Stage D disease
8. Nursing interventions for screening, detection, and prevention
      a. Recommend a rectal examination every year for all men under age 50 and every 6 months for men age 50 and older
      b. Refer the patient for medical evaluation if signs and symptoms of prostatic cancer develop
9. Nursing interventions for psychosocial needs
      a. Encourage the patient to express feelings regarding diagnosis, treatment plan, and the possible impact of disease on his life-style
      b. Assess patient and family coping mechanisms
      c. Determine the availability of support resources and help the patient gain access to appropriate resources.
      d. Promote open communication between the patient and family
      e. Provide emotional support for a patient concerned about loss of sexual function and urinary continence

10. Surgical interventions
    a. Surgery may be used alone or in combination with other treatments
    b. Radical prostatectomy, involving resection of the entire prostate, the seminal vesicles, and a portion of the bladder neck, can cure prostatic cancer
    c. Radical prostatectomy causes impotence in approximately 90% of patients
    d. Radical retropubic prostatectomy allows for lymph node dissection and results in better urinary control and less stricture formation
    e. Radical perineal prostatectomy affords a better view of the bladder neck during surgery but does not allow for lymph node dissection
    f. Transurethral resection (TUR) and open enucleation are performed to remove obstructions, which palliates symptoms
    g. TUR destroys the internal bladder sphincter, which often results in retrograde ejaculation of semen during orgasm. Although this condition does not affect the physiologic mechanisms of penile erection and orgasm, it may have an adverse psychological impact on sexual function
11. Nursing interventions for patients undergoing surgery
    a. Provide general nursing care measures applicable to all patients undergoing surgery (see Section II.B)
    b. Maintain urinary catheter patency for drainage and irrigation; monitor color of urinary drainage
    c. Assess for signs and symptoms of bleeding and shock; alert the physician if frank bleeding occurs
    d. Closely monitor intake and output and intervene as necessary to maintain fluid balance
    e. Provide pain control measures for pain resulting from surgery and bladder spasms
    f. Prevent stress on suture lines from continuous, prolonged traction of the drainage tube against the bladder
    g. Use aseptic technique during wound and catheter care to prevent infection and sepsis
    h. After radical perineal prostatectomy, provide meticulous perineal wound care to prevent infection
    i. Apply sterile dressings to perineal drain sites; use a T-binder to hold dressings in place
    j. After drain removal, provide heat lamp treatments, as ordered, to promote healing and sitz baths for cleansing and comfort
    k. Teach the patient and family how to prevent thrombus formation by performing leg exercises, wearing antiembolism stockings, or using pneumatic leg compression
    l. Inform the patient and family that incontinence affects approximately 15% of prostate surgery patients
    m. Explain that urinary dribbling is common after catheter removal
    n. Teach the patient perineal muscle exercises to help control incontinence

o. After radical perineal prostatectomy, caution the patient against using rectal tubes, rectal thermometers, suppositories, or enemas until healing is complete

12. Radiotherapeutic interventions

a. External beam radiation therapy (RT) is used as a primary therapy when cancer is localized or limited to the immediate vicinity of the prostate gland (Stages A2, B, C) or when radical prostatectomy is contraindicated or undesirable

b. External beam RT also is used as an adjuvant therapy to treat persistent residual disease following prostatic resection

c. External beam RT also is used to palliate symptoms of metastatic disease

d. External beam RT causes impotence in 30% to 50% of patients

e. Interstitial radioactive gold (^{198}Au) and radioactive iodine (^{125}I) implants also are used to treat prostatic cancer

f. Interstitial implants preserve sexual function in approximately 80% of patients; however, implants may perforate the urethra, seminal vesicles, or rectum, leading to wound infection at these sites

13. Nursing interventions for patients receiving RT

a. Provide general nursing care measures applicable to all patients receiving RT (see section II.C)

b. Assess for and intervene as necessary to control cystitis and proctitis

c. Maintain a fluid intake of at least 1 liter/day to help prevent urinary retention

d. Monitor intake and output and intervene as necessary to maintain fluid balance

e. Administer analgesics for pain as needed and as ordered

f. Administer antispasmodics, as ordered, to alleviate bladder spasms

g. Administer antidiarrheal agents, as ordered

h. Promote a low-residue diet to decrease stool frequency

i. Administer steroid suppositories and enemas, as ordered, to reduce inflammation

j. Provide meticulous perianal skin care to help prevent infection

k. When caring for a patient with interstitial implants, carefully check linens and urine for dislodged implant material; keep all linens in the patients room until they have been checked by radiation safety personnel

l. Minimize exposure of yourself and others to a patient with implants

m. Reassure a patient with implants that he will no longer be radioactive once the substance decays

n. Discuss when the patient may resume sexual activity

14. Chemotherapeutic interventions

a. Chemotherapy is used as palliative treatment when hormonal therapy fails

b. Both single-agent and combination chemotherapy are used

15. Nursing interventions for patients receiving chemotherapy for prostate cancer are similar to those for all patients receiving chemotherapy (see Section II.D)

16. Hormonal therapeutic interventions
    a. Hormonal therapy aims to palliate symptoms of metastatic disease
    b. Response rate to hormonal therapy is high, although the effect on survival rate is unknown
    c. Hormonal therapy for prostatic cancer involves interventions to prevent or inhibit androgen formation or use, such as administering estrogen (diethylstilbestrol) to block release of leutinizing hormone from the pituitary; orchiectomy to remove the primary source of testosterone; medical adrenalectomy to remove secondary sources of testosterone; administering drugs such as cyproterone and flutamide to interfere with cellular androgen activity; and hypophysectomy to remove pituitary control
17. Nursing interventions for patients receiving hormonal therapy
    a. Teach the patient and family about interventions, possible adverse effects, and goals of treatment
    b. Monitor a patient receiving diethylstilbestrol for sodium and fluid retention, hypercalcemia, hypertension, feminization, gynecomastia, and impotence and loss of libido
    c. Provide routine postoperative care following orchiectomy
    d. Reassure the patient that orchiectomy does not cause adverse effects such as feminization, gynecomastia, or voice change

C. Testicular cancer
1. General information
   a. About 97% of all testicular tumors form in germinal tissue
   b. Testicular tumors of germinal origin include include seminomas (also called germinomas) and nonseminomas
   c. Seminomas may be typical or atypical. They usually are large tumors involving only minimal hemorrhage and necrosis, and occur most commonly in patients with cryptorchidism
   d. Seminomas account for 40% to 50% of testicular germ cell cancers and occur in men over age 30
   e. Nonseminomas include embryonal carcinomas, teratomas, choriocarcinomas, and yolk sac tumors
   f. Embryonal carcinomas and teratomas are usually bulky and grow rapidly, causing areas of necrosis and hemorrhage
   g. Embryonal carcinomas and teratomas account for approximately 50% of testicular cancers, occurring primarily in men between ages 20 and 30
   h. Yolk sac tumors typically occur in children
   i. Approximately 3% of testicular tumors form in stromal tissue; types include interstitial cell tumors (Leydig cell tumors) and gonadal-stromal tumors
2. Epidemiology
   a. Testicular cancer accounts for only 1% to 2% of all cancer in men, but is the most common malignancy in men between ages 20 and 40
   b. Testicular cancer causes less than 0.5% of male cancer deaths

  c. Incidence is three times higher in whites than in blacks

  d. Scandinavian countries report the highest incidence worldwide

3. Risk factors

  a. Cryptorchidism (increases risk to 3 to 14 times normal)

  b. Maternal use of exogenous estrogen during pregnancy

4. Clinical manifestations

  a. Painless testicular enlargement or mass

  b. Acute epididymitis

  c. Gynecomastia

  d. Infertility

  e. Back pain

  f. Abdominal mass

  g. Cough (if lung metastasis has occurred)

5. Diagnostic tests

  a. Radical inguinal orchiectomy for biopsy

  b. Immunologic assays, including serum alpha-fetoprotein (α-FP), serum human chorionic gonadotropin (HCG), and urinary HCG

6. Staging

  a. Testicular cancer is staged using the TNM system of classification or other staging systems based on lymph node involvement

  b. Procedures used in staging include chest X-ray, chest tomography or CT scan, lymphangiography, abdominal CT scan, abdominal ultrasonography, and IVP

7. Natural progression of disease

  a. Routes of metastasis include lymphatic spread and hematogenous spread

  b. Sites of metastasis include lymph nodes, bone, lungs, liver, and brain

  c. Prognosis: testicular cancer survival rate has improved significantly as a result of the use of serum tumor markers such as α-FP and beta-HCG to identify disease and evaluate effectiveness of treatment. Five-year survival rate for patients with seminomas range from 96.4% for Stage A disease to 77.8% for Stage C disease. Five-year survival rate for patients with nonseminomas range from 100% for Stage A disease to 50% for Stage C disease

8. Nursing interventions for screening, detection, and prevention

  a. Teach patients how to perform a testicular self-examination and encourage them to do so monthly

  b. Encourage parents to have a child's cryptorchidism corrected as early as possible

  c. Encourage a patient with signs and symptoms of testicular cancer to seek prompt medical evaluation

9. Nursing interventions for psychosocial needs

  a. Encourage the patient to express feelings about the diagnosis, treatment plan, and impact of disease on his life-style

  b. Assess patient and family coping mechanisms

  c. Promote open communication between the patient and family

    d. Provide emotional support for a patient concerned about possible alteration in sexual function and identity

    e. Provide fertility counseling, as necessary; e.g., explain the option of depositing semen in a sperm bank before orchiectomy for subsequent use in artificial insemination

    f. As appropriate, discuss the possible use of a testicular prosthesis with the patient

10. Surgical interventions

    a. Radical inguinal orchiectomy is considered diagnostic and curative

    b. This procedure involves removal of the testis, epididymis, portions of the vas deferens, and associated lymphatics and blood vessels

    c. Radical inguinal orchiectomy may compromise fertility even though erectile ability remains unaffected

    d. Retroperitoneal lymphadenectomy is used to stage and debulk non-seminomatous germ cell tumors; this procedure is performed only after radiography shows evidence of lymph node involvement (positive nodes indicate the need for chemotherapy)

    e. Retroperitoneal lymphadenectomy may interfere with sympathetic nerve supply, causing ejaculatory dysfunction and sterility; erectile ability remains unaffected, however

11. Nursing interventions for patients undergoing surgery

    a. Provide general nursing care measures applicable to all patients undergoing surgery (see section II.B)

    b. Assess hemodynamic status for signs of hemorrhage and shock

    c. Check incisional dressings for signs of bleeding

    d. Use aseptic technique for dressing changes to prevent infection

    e. Counsel the patient regarding possible changes in sexual identity and function

    f. Inform the patient that retroperitoneal lymphadenectomy may cause an inability to ejaculate, but reassure him that his ability to experience erection and orgasm will be unaffected

12. Radiotherapeutic interventions

    a. RT has proven highly effective in treating seminomas

    b. Radiographic examination revealing negative retroperitoneal lymph nodes calls for irradiation of retroperitoneal lymph nodes only

    c. Positive retroperitoneal lymph nodes calls for irradiation of the mediastinum and supraclavicular areas

    d. RT is not commonly used to treat nonseminomas because of the usual effectiveness of chemotherapy in this application

13. Nursing interventions for patients receiving RT

    a. Provide general nursing care measures applicable to all patients receiving RT (see Section II.C)

    b. Shield the unaffected testis to help preserve fertility

    c. Inform the patient that spermatogenesis may be affected even with shielding

d. Explain the usual recovery time required for resumption of spermatogenesis. Sperm count should return to pretreatment level within 9 to 12 months after treatment with doses of 100 rad, within 30 months with doses of 200 rad, and within 5 years with doses of 600 rad or more

14. Chemotherapeutic interventions
    a. Chemotherapy is not indicated for early Stage A or Stage B seminomas
    b. The Einhorn regimen of cisplatin, vinblastine, and bleomycin (PVB) has proven effective in treating nonseminomatous germ cell cancers and disseminated seminomas
    c. Chemotherapy to treat nonseminomas is indicated when radiologic evidence of retroperitoneal disease exists; when lymph node dissection provides histologic evidence of retroperitoneal disease; when elevated tumor markers (beta-HCG, α-FP) persist for one month after orchiectomy; or if cancer recurs
    d. Salvage chemotherapy is used if the patient demonstrates incomplete response or relapse

15. Nursing interventions for patients receiving chemotherapy
    a. Provide general nursing care measures applicable to all patients receiving chemotherapy (see Section II.D)
    b. Keep in mind that the Einhorn regimen of PVB is highly toxic; closely assess for leukopenia and sepsis
    c. Provide thorough patient education, emotional support, and adequate management of adverse effects to help ensure patient compliance with therapy

D. Breast cancer

1. General information
    a. Many types of breast cancer exist
    b. Infiltrating intraductal carcinoma is the most common histologic type, accounting for 75% to 78% of all breast cancers
    c. Histologic type does not influence choice of primary treatment for breast cancer, except in inflammatory breast carcinoma
    d. Common sites of breast cancer include the upper outer quadrant of the breast and under the nipple
    e. The trend in breast cancer treatment is toward a two-step procedure of biopsy for diagnosis followed by mastectomy, if indicated, at a later date
    f. Advanced disease calls for a multimodal approach to treatment

2. Epidemiology
    a. Each year, 114,000 women are diagnosed with breast cancer in the United States; 33% of these women eventually die as a result of breast cancer
    b. Breast cancer is the second-leading cause of cancer death for women (after lung cancer) in the United States

   c. In the western hemisphere, 1 in 11 women will develop breast cancer at some point in her life

   d. Incidence increases with age, peaking between ages 50 and 59, then declines after menopause

   e. Developed regions of the world, such as North America, northwestern Europe, Australia, and New Zealand, report the highest incidences

3. Risk factors

   a. Family history of breast cancer (increases risk to 2 or 3 times normal)

   b. Family history of premenopausal bilateral breast cancer (increases risk to 7 or 8 times normal)

   c. History of cancer in opposite breast

   d. Onset of early menarche

   e. First pregnancy after age 30

   f. Late menopause

   g. Nulliparity

   h. Obesity

   i. High dietary fat intake

   j. History of fibrocystic breast disease

   k. History of radiation exposure

4. Clinical manifestations

   a. Painless lump or thickening in breast

   b. Nipple retraction or elevation

   c. Breast tissue dimpling or retraction (peau d'orange)

   d. Edema of breast

   e. Breast tissue or nipple ulceration

   f. Nipple discharge

   g. Firm, enlarged axillary nodes

   h. Pathologic fracture resulting from bone metastasis

5. Diagnostic tests

   a. Mammography

   b. Biopsy and histopathologic examination, which may include percutaneous needle biopsy, needle aspiration of cystic fluid, and excisional or incisional biopsies

6. Staging

   a. The TNM system is used to stage breast cancer

   b. Procedures used in staging include mammography, biopsy, chest X-ray, CBC and blood chemistries, bone scan, and liver scan (if indicated by physical assessment findings or liver function tests)

7. Natural progression of disease

   a. Routes of metastasis include direct extension, lymphatic spread with primary drainage to ipsilateral axillary nodes, and hematogenous spread

   b. Sites of metastasis include regional lymph nodes, lungs, bone, liver, and brain

    c. Prognosis: Difficulties in treating breast cancer stem from the inability to affect occult metastases that manifest later in remote sites. Because breast cancer may recur 5 to 20 years or more after treatment, a patient free from disease for 5 years cannot be considered cured. Five-year survival rate ranges from 85% for Stage I disease to 10% for Stage IV disease

8. Nursing interventions for screening, detection, and prevention
   a. Teach patients the importance of decreasing dietary fat intake, and provide information on how to do so
   b. Teach patients about early clinical manifestations of breast cancer
   c. Teach patients how to perform a breast self-examination and urge them to do so monthly
   d. Discuss American Cancer Society mammogram guidelines with patients, and recommend a baseline mammogram for all patients between ages 35 and 40 and an annual mammogram for patients at risk and all patients age 40 and older

9. Nursing interventions for psychosocial needs
   a. Encourage the patient to express feelings about the cancer, its treatment plan, and the expected impact on her life-style
   b. Evaluate the patient's feelings regarding the importance of her breasts to her sexual identity, relationships, and body-image
   c. Promote patient understanding of treatment options, such as lumpectomy and mastectomy
   d. Assess patient and family coping mechanisms
   e. Determine the availability of support resources and help the patient gain access to appropriate resources
   f. Promote open communication between the patient and her family or partner
   g. Discuss possible options for breast reconstruction, such as the use of implants or muscle flaps
   h. Refer the patient to appropriate support groups, such as I Can Cope, Reach to Recovery, and AFTER (Ask a Friend To Explain Reconstruction)

10. Surgical interventions
    a. Cure rates are good for primary surgical treatment in local disease without nodal spread
    b. Modified radical mastectomy (also known as total mastectomy with axillary dissection), a standard treatment for Stage I and Stage II disease, involves en bloc resection of breast tissue, pectoralis minor muscles, and intervening lymphatics and axillary lymph nodes
    c. Radical mastectomy, a rarely used procedure, involves resection of the tissues removed in modified radical mastectomy plus the pectoralis major muscle
    d. Survival and recurrence rates are equal for radical mastectomy and modified radical mastectomy; modified radical mastectomy causes less mutilation

      e. Partial mastectomy followed by RT is used for tumors less than 2 cm (¾″) in diameter

      f. Survival and recurrence rates for partial mastectomy with RT are similar to those for modified radical mastectomy

      g. Tylectomy (lumpectomy) followed by RT is used to resect gross tumors

      h. Survival rate for tylectomy with RT is currently under investigation

      i. Mastectomy may be indicated in a patient with advanced, extensive local disease with no evidence of remote metastasis

11. Nursing interventions for patients undergoing surgery

      a. Provide general nursing care measures applicable to all patients undergoing surgery (see Section II.B)

      b. Determine the patient's knowledge of breast cancer and her previous experiences with the disease

      c. Teach the patient how to perform permitted arm and shoulder range-of-motion exercises 2 to 7 days after surgery

      d. Encourage constant arm elevation to decrease lymphedema

      e. Avoid trauma to the arm on the affected side—such as injections, venipunctures, and blood pressure monitoring—to prevent lymphedema and other complications of impaired circulation after surgery

      f. Promote good skin and nail care to help prevent infection and other complications of impaired circulation after surgery

      g. Teach the patient how to use a pressure sleeve to help prevent lymphedema

12. Radiotherapeutic interventions

      a. Survival and recurrence rates are comparable for RT used alone and RT used after mastectomy

      b. Primary therapy with RT typically involves external beam irradiation to the breast and the ipsilateral mammary, supraclavicular, and axillary lymph nodes, followed by implantation of ^{192}Ir into the biopsy area and 2 cm (¾″) of surrounding tissue to provide additional radiation

      c. RT also may be effective as an adjuvant treatment following partial mastectomy or lumpectomy

      d. RT followed by chemotherapy may be used to treat inflammatory breast cancer

      e. RT also may be used to treat local recurrences when massive axillary nodes do not respond to systemic treatment, to ablate ovarian function and remove endogenous sources of estrogen, and to palliate symptoms of metastatic disease

13. Nursing interventions for patients receiving RT

      a. Provide general nursing care measures applicable to all patients receiving RT (see Section II.C)

      b. Assess the patient's knowledge of and previous experience with breast cancer and RT; correct any misconceptions and fill in knowledge gaps

      c. Teach the patient how to perform arm and shoulder range-of-motion exercises, as appropriate, to maintain function

    d. Avoid trauma to the arm on the affected side

    e. Encourage the patient to elevate her arm and to use pressure sleeves to prevent or minimize lymphedema after irradiation of axillary nodes

14. Chemotherapeutic interventions

    a. Chemotherapy may be used as an adjunct to surgical treatment to inhibit relapse and prolong survival rate in Stage II disease, for estrogen receptor (ER)-negative tumors and for ER-positive tumors that no longer respond to hormonal therapy

    b. Combination chemotherapy is more effective than single-agent therapy

    c. Response to combination chemotherapy typically persists for 9 to 12 months

    d. Effective combinations include cyclophosphamide, methotrexate, and 5-fluorouracil (CMF) with or without prednisone; and cyclophosphamide, adriamycin, and 5-fluorouracil

15. Nursing interventions for patients receiving chemotherapy

    a. Provide general nursing care measures applicable to all patients receiving chemotherapy (see Section II.D)

    b. Assess the patient's knowledge of and previous experience with chemotherapy; correct misconceptions and fill in knowledge gaps

    c. Keep in mind that chemotherapy should not be administered in the same arm where RT or surgical excision of the axillary lymph nodes has been performed

16. Hormonal therapeutic interventions

    a. These interventions involve manipulation of estrogen sources through surgery, RT, or chemotherapy

    b. Hormonal interventions are indicated in metastatic disease involving an ER-positive tumor that cannot be reasonably controlled by surgery or RT

    c. Specific hormonal interventions include estrogen therapy in postmenopausal women, androgen therapy, corticosteroid therapy, anti-estrogen therapy, surgical or RT-induced castration, and medical adrenalectomy

17. Nursing interventions for patients receiving hormonal therapy

    a. As appropriate, provide general nursing care measures applicable to all patients receiving RT or chemotherapy, or undergoing surgery (see Section II)

    b. Assess the patient's knowledge of and experience with any aspect of hormonal therapy, and provide appropriate patient teaching

E. Cervical cancer

1. General information

    a. Cervical cancer often occurs at the squamo-columnar junction or transformation zone of the cervix

    b. More than 90% of cervical cancers are squamous cell cancers

    c. Approximately 5% of cervical cancers are adenocarcinomas

SQUAMOCOLUMNAR JUNCTION

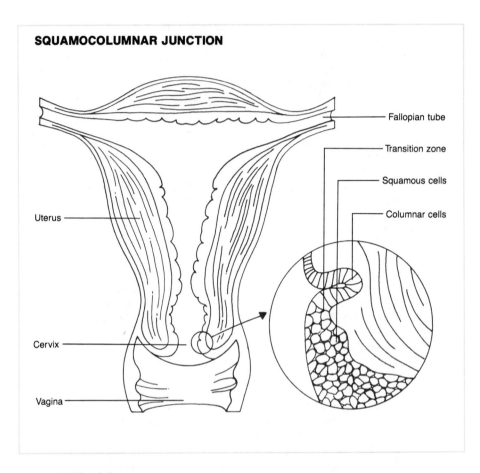

2. Epidemiology
   a. Cervical cancer is the second most common gynecologic malignancy
   b. Each year in the United States, 12,900 new cases of invasive cervical cancer are diagnosed and 7,000 women die of cervical cancer
   c. Incidence has decreased by about 50% since the advent of the Pap test in 1945
3. Risk factors
   a. Frequent sexual activity at an early age
   b. History of multiple sexual partners
   c. History of human papilloma virus infection
   d. History of herpes simplex virus type 2 infection

4. Clinical manifestations
   a. Thin, watery, blood-tinged vaginal discharge
   b. Postcoital spotting or bleeding
   c. Metrorrhagia (intermittent, painless intermenstrual bleeding)
   d. Menorrhagia (heavy or prolonged menstrual flow)
   e. Presence of exophytic, endophytic, ulcerative, or excavating lesions upon pelvic examination
   f. Pain in the pelvis, leg, or back (late symptom)
   g. Edema in the lower legs and feet (late sign)
   h. Vaginal hemorrhage (late sign)
5. Diagnostic tests
   a. Endocervical curettage
   b. Cervical biopsy
   c. Cone biopsy
6. Staging
   a. Cervical cancer is staged using the International Federation of Gynecology and Obstetrics (FIGO) system of classification, based on clinical evaluation of the lesion
   b. Procedures used in staging include examination under anesthesia, cystoscopy, proctoscopy, CBC and blood chemistries, chest X-ray, IVP, and barium enema
7. Natural progression of disease
   a. Routes of metastasis include direct extension to contiguous organs, orderly lymphatic spread, and hematogenous dissemination
   b. Common sites of metastasis include parametrium, lymph nodes, bladder, rectum, lungs, liver, and bone
   c. Prognosis based on 5-year survival rate ranges from 90% to 100% for Stage Ia disease to 5% to 10% for Stage IV disease
8. Nursing interventions for screening, detection, and prevention: Encourage annual Pap tests for all women beginning at age 18, or sooner if sexually active
9. Nursing interventions for psychosocial needs
   a. Help the patient and her family deal with anxiety and fear associated with possible loss of fertility, altered sexual function and self-image, and the possibility of death
   b. Counsel a patient who expresses guilt about the possible link between her cancer and a history of sexual promiscuity
   c. Evaluate patient and family coping mechanisms and the availability of support systems
10. Surgical interventions
    a. Surgical intervention is influenced by various factors, including the patient's age, desire to preserve reproductive or sexual function, and history of pelvic or bowel disease
    b. Surgery for preinvasive cervical disease is 100% curative; options include cryotherapy, CO_2 laser surgery, and cervical conization

     c. Surgery is the preferred treatment modality for Stage Ia and Stage Ib early invasive disease; types used include total abdominal hysterectomy (TAH), radical hysterectomy, and bilateral pelvic lymphadenectomy

     d. Radical hysterectomy may lead to complications resulting from extensive dissection near the ureters, bladder, rectum, and blood vessels

11. Nursing interventions for patients undergoing surgery

     a. Provide general nursing care measures applicable to all patients undergoing surgery (see Section II.B)

     b. Administer a preoperative vaginal douche, as ordered

     c. Monitor for signs and symptoms of bleeding; check vital signs and pad count

     d. Assess the character and amount of postoperative vaginal discharge

     e. Evaluate and record the type and amount of discharge from peritoneal cavity drainage tubes

     f. Monitor intake and output and intervene as necessary to maintain fluid balance

     g. Inform the patient and family that bladder dysfunction may continue for weeks or months after radical hysterectomy

     h. Explain that a suprapubic or urethral catheter or intermittent self-catheterization may be needed for urinary drainage until normal bladder function returns; provide patient teaching for catheterization and catheter care

     i. Teach the patient and family how to care for skin around urinary drainage site to prevent infection

     j. As appropriate, teach the patient bladder training exercises, such as intermittent clamping and release of urinary catheters to allow bladder distention and emptying

     k. Instruct the patient to avoid vaginal manipulation, such as intercourse, douching, or tampon use for 4 to 6 weeks following surgery

     l. Instruct the patient to comply with scheduled medical follow-up

12. Radiotherapeutic interventions

     a. External beam RT may be used to treat all stages of cervical cancer or to palliate symptoms caused by advanced disease

     b. External beam RT usually involves pelvic irradiation with a maximum dose of 4,500 to 5,000 rad, which is the limit of bladder and rectum tissue tolerance

     c. Internal implants are used to treat in Stage I through Stage IV disease; this therapy enables delivery of a higher maximum radiation dose to the cervix (an additional 3,000 rad) and minimizes effects on surrounding organs

     d. Implant placement is performed in the operating room with the patient under anesthesia; radiation therapist stipulates duration of implantation

13. Nursing interventions for patients receiving RT

     a. Provide general nursing care measures applicable to all patients receiving RT (see Section II.C)

      b. Inform the patient and family that proctitis and cystitis may follow external beam RT; explain signs and symptoms to watch for

      c. Inform the patient about the possibility of pelvic alopecia

      d. Provide emotional support for the patient and family

      e. Teach the patient and family appropriate safety measures for radioactive implant therapy

      f. Administer a cleansing enema, as ordered, to empty the bowel before implantation begins

      g. Assist with a pre-implant antibacterial vaginal douche, as ordered

      h. Apply antiembolism stockings before implantation to help prevent possible thrombus formation

      i. Provide a low-residue diet before implantation and while the implant is in place to decrease bowel motility

      j. As ordered, administer medications, such as diphenoxylate, to decrease bowel motility

      k. Provide urinary catheter care to prevent infection

      l. Assess for signs and symptoms of bleeding

      m. Administer anticoagulant agents, as ordered, to decrease the risk of thrombus formation

  14. Chemotherapeutic interventions

      a. Chemotherapy alone is used only as a secondary treatment for persistent or recurring cancer

      b. Response rate for single-agent chemotherapy ranges from 4% to 40%

      c. Combination chemotherapy produces a response rate ranging from 28% to 89%

      d. The median duration of response is several months

      e. Use of such agents as cisplatin, 5-fluorouracil, and hydroxyurea as radiosensitizers with RT to treat bulky tumors and advanced disease is under investigation

  15. Nursing interventions for patients receiving chemotherapy

      a. Provide general nursing care measures applicable for all patients receiving chemotherapy (see Section II.D)

      b. Provide emotional support as disease advances

F. Endometrial cancer

  1. General information

      a. Endometrial cancer is the most common gynecologic cancer

      b. Incidence has increased over the past 20 years

      c. Endometrial cancer usually is detected in early stages because of symptoms, such as vaginal bleeding

      d. Adenocarcinomas account for more than 90% of endometrial cancers

      e. Other endometrial malignancies include sarcomas and lymphomas

  2. Epidemiology

      a. Cancer of the uterus (cervix and endometrium) accounts for 10% of all cancers in American women and about 4% of all female cancer deaths in the United States

    b. Each year in the United States, 34,000 new cases of endometrial cancer are diagnosed and 3,000 women die from endometrial cancer

    c. Endometrial cancer occurs primarily in postmenopausal women, with peak incidence between ages 50 and 59

3. Risk factors
   a. Obesity
   b. Nulliparity
   c. Late menopause
   d. Hypertension
   e. Diabetes
   f. History of breast cancer
   g. History of ovarian cancer
   h. Prolonged use of estrogens
   i. Infertility
   j. Irregular menses
   k. Anovulation
   l. History of adenomatous hyperplasia
   m. Concomitant obesity, nulliparity, and late menopause (increases risk to 5 times normal)

4. Clinical manifestations
   a. Postmenopausal bleeding
   b. New onset of irregular or heavy menstrual flow
   c. Yellow or serosanguinous vaginal discharge
   d. Pyometra
   e. Lumbosacral, hypogastric, or pelvic pain

5. Diagnostic tests
   a. Pelvic examination
   b. Endometrial biopsy
   c. Fractional dilatation and curettage
   d. Pap test (may occasionally be diagnostic)

6. Staging
   a. Staging of endometrial cancer usually follows the FIGO staging system; based on clinical findings
   b. Procedures used in staging include chest X-ray, IVP, CBC, blood chemistries, and examination under anesthesia (EUA)
   c. Less commonly used staging procedures include barium enema, cystoscopy, proctoscopy, CT scans, and lymphangiography

7. Natural progression of disease
   a. Routes of metastasis include direct extension, lymphatic spread, and hematogenous spread
   b. Sites of metastasis include lungs, liver, bone, brain, vagina, peritoneal cavity, and omentum
   c. Prognosis is based on numerous factors, including cell type, disease stage and grade, uterine size, myometrial and peritoneal invasion, lymph node involvement, and adnexal metastasis; 5-year survival rate ranges from 72% for Stage I disease to 9% for Stage IV disease

8. Nursing interventions for screening, detection, and prevention
   a. Inform patients that postmenopausal bleeding always warrants further investigation for possible endometrial cancer
   b. Refer patients with possible signs and symptoms of endometrial cancer for further medical evaluation
   c. As appropriate, teach patients the importance of using progestin therapy along with necessary estrogen replacement therapy to reduce the risk of chronic unopposed estrogen exposure
   d. Encourage obese patients to lose weight
   e. Teach patients with adenomatous hyperplasia about the importance of treatment and regular follow-ups to prevent cancer
9. Nursing interventions for psychosocial needs
   a. Encourage the patient and her partner to discuss their feelings regarding possible consequences of the disease and its treatment, such as loss of fertility, disruption of sexual function, mutilation, or death
   b. Encourage the patient to express feelings about the disease's effect on her sense of femininity, sexual identity, body image, and self-esteem
   c. Promote open communication between the patient and family
10. Surgical interventions
    a. Surgery for Stage I and Stage II disease usually involves total abdominal hysterectomy–bilateral salpingo-oophorectomy (TAH-BSO), pelvic and para-aortic lymph node dissection, and peritoneal cytology
    b. The need for and direction of further treatment is determined by pathologic findings
    c. Stage I, grade 1 disease with no disease outside the uterus requires no further treatment; Stage I disease with high-grade tumors, disease involving the myometrium, or disease extending beyond the uterus usually requires further treatment
    d. Stage III and Stage IV disease are uncommon and require individualized treatment
11. Nursing interventions for patients undergoing surgery
    a. Provide general nursing care measures applicable to all patients undergoing surgery (see Section II.B)
    b. Before surgery, administer a cleansing enema and a vaginal douche with antiseptic solution, as ordered
    c. After surgery, assess cardiopulmonary status; monitor vital signs for abnormalities
    d. Help the patient turn, cough, and deep-breathe every 2 hours to prevent pulmonary complications
    e. Inspect the abdominal wound and dressing for signs of bleeding, infection, or improper healing
    f. Assess function of nasogastric tube, if present, and monitor color and amount of drainage
    g. Assess quality and quantity of discharge from drainage sites
    h. Encourage the patient to walk as soon as possible after surgery to prevent thrombus formation

     i. Inform the patient that vaginal discharge is normal and should be pink-tinged; instruct the patient to notify physician if drainage increases or changes color

     j. Instruct the patient to avoid vaginal manipulation, such as intercourse, douching, or tampon use, until wound healing is complete

     k. Tell the patient to report any abnormal pain, fever, bleeding, and nausea or vomiting

     l. Inform premenopausal patients that BSO may induce symptoms of menopause, such as hot flashes; intervene as necessary to help alleviate symptoms

12. Radiotherapeutic interventions
    a. RT may be the primary treatment for Stage I and Stage II disease in patients who are not surgical candidates; often used in advanced disease
    b. RT may be used for Stage II disease before hysterectomy, to shrink tumors and provide greater surgical margins
    c. Postoperative RT may be used as an adjuvant therapy for Stage II disease
    d. Intracavitary radiation may be used with external beam RT to maximize radiation dosage and minimize effects on surrounding tissue

13. Nursing interventions for patients receiving RT
    a. Provide general nursing care measures applicable to all patients receiving RT (see Section II.C)
    b. After RT, instruct the patient to avoid vaginal manipulation until the physician allows
    c. Also after RT, encourage the patient to use a water-based vaginal lubricant to increase comfort during intercourse

14. Chemotherapeutic interventions
    a. Single-agent and combination chemotherapy are used to treat Stage III and Stage IV disease
    b. Response rate for chemotherapy ranges from 30% to 50%
    c. Agents used include doxorubicin, cisplatin, melphalan, 5-fluorouracil and cyclophosphamide
    d. Hormonal therapy is used to treat advanced and recurring disease
    e. Response rate for hormonal therapy is about 33%; response is related to tumor grade
    f. Hormonal agents used include medroxyprogesterone acetate and megestrol acetate
    g. Researchers are investigating the use and manipulation of estrogen and progesterone receptors to predict and improve treatment response

15. Nursing interventions for patients receiving chemotherapy
    a. Provide general nursing care measures applicable for all patients receiving chemotherapy (see Section II.D)
    b. Explain the actions of and reasons for using specific chemotherapeutic and hormonal agents
    c. Point out possible minor adverse reactions to hormonal therapy, such as fluid retention, increased appetite, weight gain, and slightly increased risk of thrombosis

G. Ovarian cancer
1. General information
    a. Ovarian cancer often is asymptomatic until late stages
    b. Early diagnosis is made difficult by the typically vague symptoms
    c. Epithelial cancers account for 90% of ovarian malignancies
    d. Ovarian cancer is considered a disease of the peritoneal cavity because the tumor cells derive from the same embryonic tissue as that of the peritoneal cavity and the disease commonly extends to the peritoneal cavity
    e. Death usually results from complications of intra-abdominal tumor dissemination, such as carcinomatosis ileus, malabsorption, intestinal obstruction, electrolyte imbalance, sepsis, or cardiovascular collapse
2. Epidemiology
    a. Ovarian cancer accounts for 4% of all cancers in women in the United States, and is the fourth-leading cause of cancer death in women
    b. Each year in the United States, 19,000 new cases of ovarian cancer are diagnosed and 12,000 women die of ovarian cancer
    c. Women between ages 40 and 65 are at greatest risk
    d. Peak incidence occurs between ages 50 and 60
    e. Incidence is highest in highly industrialized countries
    f. A history of oral contraceptive use or pregnancy may reduce the risk of ovarian cancer
3. Risk factors
    a. Nulliparity
    b. Infertility
    c. Habitation in an industrialized country
    d. History of breast cancer
    e. History of colon cancer
    f. Exposure to talc
4. Clinical manifestations
    a. Palpable abdominal mass
    b. Ascites
    c. Dyspepsia
    d. Urinary frequency
    e. Vague abdominal discomfort
    f. Mild GI dysfunction
5. Diagnostic tests
    a. Pelvic examination
    b. Pelvic ultrasonography
    c. Barium enema
    d. IVP
6. Staging
    a. Staging of ovarian cancer uses the FIGO staging system based on surgical and pathologic findings, not on clinical findings

      b. Procedures used in staging include staging laparotomy (the preferred choice for diagnosis, staging, and treatment—provides definitive diagnosis), chest X-ray, abdominal and pelvic ultrasonography, CT scan, and proctosigmoidoscopy

7. Natural progression of disease
      a. Routes of metastasis include intraperitoneal seeding, direct extension, lymphatic spread, and hematogenous spread
      b. Common sites of metastasis include peritoneal surfaces of abdominal and pelvic organs, such as fallopian tubes, uterus, bladder, rectosigmoid colon, peritoneum, liver, diaphragm, and lymphatic channels
      c. Prognosis is based on 5-year survival rate for each disease stage, which ranges from 70% for Stage I disease to 0% for Stage IV disease

8. Nursing interventions for screening, detection, and prevention
      a. Keep in mind that prevention is not feasible because causative factors remain unknown
      b. Inform patients that vague abdominal discomfort could be an early sign of ovarian cancer—especially in women ages 50 to 65. Encourage patients with vague abdominal symptoms to seek further medical evaluation
      c. Encourage all women to have regular pelvic examinations to improve the chance of early disease detection
      d. Inform patients that a history of oral contraceptive use or pregnancy may decrease the risk of ovarian cancer

9. Nursing interventions for psychosocial needs
      a. Counsel a patient with ovarian cancer who feels guilty about not seeking prompt medical attention for nonspecific symptoms
      b. Allow the patient and family to express any anger they may feel toward health care professionals for failing to diagnose the disease in its early stages
      c. Encourage the patient and family to discuss their fears and anxieties regarding loss of reproductive function, loss of sexual appeal, menopause, osteoporosis, and death
      d. Evaluate the impact of diagnosis and disease on the patient's sexual identity and body image

10. Surgical interventions
      a. Laparotomy with tumor excision, the primary treatment for ovarian cancer, involves TAH-BSO, omentectomy, pelvic and para-aortic lymph node dissection, and fluid aspiration for cytology
      b. Surgical interventions aim to stage the disease, maximally debulk the tumor in preparation for adjuvant treatment, or improve prognosis by decreasing tumor burden
      c. A patient with residual disease of less than 1 cm (½″) (optimal resection) usually has a better prognosis than a patient with residual disease of greater than 1 cm (suboptimal resection)

    d. Second-look laparotomy often is performed following a complete chemotherapy regimen to evaluate disease status and plan further therapy. This procedure involves taking biopsies of peritoneum, adhesions, suspicious areas, and areas of residual tumor from the original laparotomy; obtaining cytologies; sampling para-aortic lymph nodes; and thoroughly examining intestines and all abdominal and pelvic structures

11. Nursing interventions for patients undergoing surgery
    a. Provide general nursing care measures applicable to all patients undergoing surgery (see Section II.B)
    b. Encourage early ambulation and use of antiembolism stockings to prevent thrombus formation
    c. Inspect incision and dressing for signs of wound complications
    d. Monitor drainage decompression catheters, such as nasogastric tube and urrinary catheter, for amount and character of drainage
    e. Assess color and amount of vaginal drainage; monitor pad count. Vaginal drainage should be dark brown in color; notify physician immediately of bright red drainage or saturated pads, which may indicate hemorrhage

12. Radiotherapeutic interventions
    a. External beam RT is used primarily for microscopic disease, for tumors less than 1 cm in size, and following a positive second-look laparotomy
    b. External beam RT carries a high incidence of bowel complications resulting from pelvic and abdominal irradiation
    c. Intraperitoneal administration of radioactive chromic phosphate (^{32}P) may be used following a negative second-look laparotomy or a second-look laparotomy that reveals microscopic disease, and in early Stage I and Stage II disease

13. Nursing interventions for patients receiving RT
    a. Provide general nursing care measures applicable to all patients receiving chemotherapy (see Section II.C)
    b. Monitor CBC and platelet count weekly to detect blood abnormalities
    c. Inform the patient and family that receiving ^{32}P therapy does not make her radioactive
    d. Promote an even distribution of ^{32}P in the peritoneal cavity by turning the patient regularly. As ordered, position the patient on her right side, supine, on her left side, prone, and in Trendelenburg and reverse Trendelenburg positions
    e. Explain the signs and symptoms of bowel obstruction and stress the importance of immediately reporting them
    f. Stress the need for routine follow-up examinations

14. Chemotherapeutic interventions
    a. Systemic chemotherapy, the preferred treatment following surgery, is used in Stage II through Stage IV disease and selected cases of Stage I disease
    b. Single-agent or combination chemotherapy is used, typically in multiple cycles. Advanced disease usually calls for combination chemotherapy

      c. Commonly used antineoplastic agents include cisplatin and cyclophosphamide with or without doxorubicin

      d. Response rate to chemotherapy ranges from 60% to 80%

      e. Complete clinical response—eradication of all disease traces—occurs in approximately 40% of patients receiving systemic chemotherapy

      f. Tumor debulking to 1 cm or less before chemotherapy improves patient response

      g. Intraperitoneal chemotherapy (IPC) involves administering agents directly into the peritoneal cavity using a dialysis catheter with an external catheter or an implanted port

      h. IPC prolongs tumor exposure to antineoplastic agents (because the peritoneum absorbs the drug slowly) and allows delivery of a maximum dose to the peritoneal cavity while minimizing systemic drug levels

15. Nursing interventions for patients receiving chemotherapy

      a. Provide general nursing care measures applicable to all patients receiving chemotherapy (see Section II.D)

      b. Perform catheter or access port site care in accordance with institutional policy to prevent infection

      c. Teach the patient and family the signs and symptoms of infection and measures for IPC site care

Points to Remember

Symptoms of prostate cancer often mimic symptoms of benign prostatic hypertrophy.

Inguinal orchiectomy is the procedure used to diagnose and treat testicular cancer.

Breast cancer screening relies on breast self-examination and mammography.

Use of the Pap test has resulted in decreased mortality from cervical cancer.

Treatment for endometrial cancer commonly involves total abdominal hysterectomy, bilateral salpingo-oophorectomy, and lymph node dissection with or without radiation therapy. Hormonal therapy helps control advanced and recurring endometrial cancer.

Because early symptoms rarely occur, ovarian cancer often progresses undetected until late stages of the disease.

Nursing interventions for a patient with cancer of the reproductive tract should always include psychosocial and sexual assessment and fertility counseling.

Glossary

Cryptorchidism—failure of one or both of the testes to descend from the abdomen into the scrotum

Endogenous estrogen—estrogen produced within the body rather than supplied from an outside source

Peau d'orange—condition in which skin appears dimpled, resembling the skin of an orange

Prostatism—symptom complex most commonly resulting from prostatic enlargement and involving reduced force and caliber of urinary stream, urinary hesitancy and dribbling, a sensation of incomplete bladder emptying, and possibly urinary retention

Pyometra—accumulation of pus in the uterine cavity

Spermatogenesis—development of mature spermatozoa

Transformation zone—area of the cervix in which cells change from glandular cells to squamous cells

Tylectomy—type of partial mastectomy involving removal of the tumor and some adjacent tissue in an attempt to preserve the breast

Cancer of the Hematologic System

Learning Objectives

After studying this section, the reader should be able to:

- Discuss the epidemiology and risk factors for hematologic system cancers.

- List possible clinical manifestations of each cancer.

- Identify several tests used to diagnose and stage each cancer.

- Discuss common routes of dissemination for each cancer.

- Identify several medical and surgical interventions for each cancer.

- Discuss nursing interventions for patients undergoing treatment for hematologic cancer.

XII. Cancer of the Hematologic System

A. **Introduction**
   1. Hematologic system cancers include leukemias and lymphomas
   2. Leukemias occur in the blood system, causing a proliferation of malignant white blood cells (WBC)
   3. Lymphomas occur in the lymphatic system, specifically in the lymph nodes
   4. Lymphomas are a malignant variant of the lymphocyte cell line; cancer may develop at any time during cellular development
   5. Cell maturation stops when malignant transformation occurs. After transformation, the cell will perform functions typical of its pretransformation development stage. For instance, if the cell's function at the time of malignant transformation was to secrete an antibody protein, the tumor cell will continue to secrete the antibody protein, but in abnormal quantities
   6. Lymphomas are classified as cancers of either T-lymphocytes or B-lymphocytes
   7. Lymphomas are further classified as either Hodgkin's disease (HD) or non-Hodgkin's lymphomas (NHL), and each has a unique disease progression, treatment, and prognosis

B. **Leukemia**
   1. General information
      a. The cause of leukemia is unknown
      b. In leukemia, normal cell maturation is arrested. Abnormal proliferation of immature cells crowds out normal bone marrow cells, inhibiting hematopoiesis and resulting in total replacement of the bone marrow with immature cells. Growth and function of other bone marrow elements also are inhibited
      c. Leukemia is classified according to onset as either *acute* (sudden onset and rapid disease progression) or *chronic* (asymptomatic, slower progression)
      d. Leukemia is also classified according to the predominant malignant cell and named for the point at which cellular maturation stops
      e. The four general classifications of leukemia are *acute myelogenous leukemia (AML)*; *acute lymphoblastic leukemia (ALL)*; *chronic myelogenous leukemia (CML)*; and *chronic lymphocytic leukemia (CLL)*
      f. In AML, myeloid cell line maturation stops at the myeloblast stage; cells can proliferate but cannot function and mature
      g. In AML, myeloblasts can crowd out normal bone marrow cells and infiltrate various organs, causing death from bleeding or infection in 2 to 4 weeks if not treated

BLOOD CELL DIFFERENTIATION

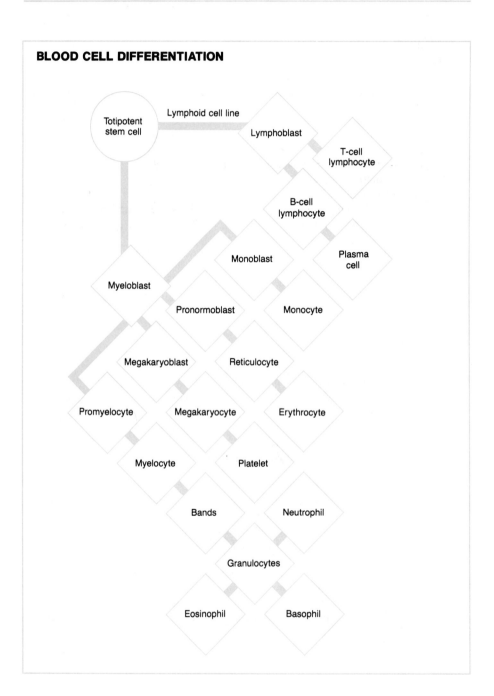

    h. In ALL, lymphoid line maturation stops at the lymphoblast stage; infiltration and proliferation in the bone marrow inhibits the function of other bone marrow elements

    i. In ALL, organ or lymph node enlargement or obstruction may cause pain; if untreated, death may occur rapidly from bleeding and infection

    j. ALL can enter sanctuary sites (areas that cytotoxic drugs fail to permeate, such as the GI system, testes, and central nervous system), resulting in relapse after disease remission

    k. CML is characterized by an abnormal proliferation of granulocytic precursors; most CML patients have the Philadelphia (Ph^1) chromosome (significance unknown), and some have splenomegaly

    l. CML has two distinct phases: a *chronic phase*, consisting of an asymptomatic pre-leukemic stage that may progress to a symptomatic active stage, and an *acute phase*, consisting of the blast crisis that invariably causes death in 3 to 6 months

    m. Death in CML usually results from infection caused by granulocyte dysfunction, chemotherapy-induced pancytopenia, embolism, or overwhelming growth of myeloblasts in the bone marrow

    n. CLL is characterized by an abnormal proliferation of early B-cell lymphocytes—aberrant mature lymphocytes that proliferate slowly and have a long life but cannot function well

    o. CLL remains asymptomatic for a long time because of a slow rate of lymphocyte growth; symptoms appear as CLL cells infiltrate the bone marrow

    p. Death in CLL usually results from infection caused by pancytopenia and hypogammaglobulinemia

2. Epidemiology

    a. Leukemia accounts for 3% of all cancers diagnosed in the United States

    b. Each year, about 26,900 Americans develop leukemia and 18,000 Americans die as a result of leukemia

    c. Incidence of leukemia increases with age—except for incidence of ALL, which is highest in children

    d. Leukemia accounts for 30% of all childhood cancers

    e. Incidence of acute leukemia in men is 50% higher than in women

    f. Incidence of chronic leukemia in men is twice that in women

3. Risk factors

    a. Genetic predispositions, such as Down's syndrome, albinism, and congenital immunodeficiency syndromes

    b. History of prolonged radiation exposure

    c. Chronic exposure to benzene

    d. Repeated exposure to certain drugs, including alkylating agents, ^{32}P, and chloramphenicol

    e. History of exposure to oncogenic viruses

4. Clinical manifestations (result from proliferation of leukocytes within the bone marrow, spleen, liver, and lymphatic system)
   a. Anemia
   b. Fatigue
   c. Pallor
   d. Bleeding
   e. Petechiae
   f. Ecchymoses
   g. Infection
   h. Fever
   i. Night sweats
   j. Pain
   k. Pancytopenia
   l. Lymphadenopathy
   m. Manifestations of specific organ involvement, such as joint swelling, headache, GI tract bleeding, pleural effusion, papilledema, retinal hemorrhage, hepatomegaly, and splenomegaly
5. Diagnostic tests
   a. Complete blood count (CBC)
   b. Bone marrow aspiration
   c. Chest X-ray
   d. Intravenous pyelography
   e. Lumbar puncture (to evaluate cerebrospinal fluid in ALL and AML)
6. Staging: No staging system is used for leukemia
7. Natural progression of disease
   a. Leukemic cells originate in the bone marrow and crowd out normal marrow cells
   b. Leukemic cells may infiltrate organs
   c. Prognosis varies with type of leukemia; death results from complications secondary to loss of normal bone marrow cells (e.g., bleeding or infection) or organ failure caused by leukemic cell infiltration
8. Nursing interventions for screening, detection, and prevention
   a. Keep in mind that no screening tests for leukemia exist
   b. Be aware of the risk factors and signs and symptoms associated with leukemia
   c. Encourage and help a patient with possible signs and symptoms of leukemia to seek prompt medical attention
9. Nursing interventions for psychosocial needs
   a. Assess the patient's and family's understanding of leukemia, the treatment plan, and possible complications
   b. Assess patient and family coping mechanisms
   c. Determine the availability of support resources and help the patient gain access to appropriate resources
   d. Encourage the patient to express feelings about the diagnosis, treatment plan, and impact of the disease on his life-style

e. Help the patient and family adjust to the long-term nature of the disease and its treatment

f. Help the patient cope with the periods of protective isolation and extensive tests and procedures required for patient protection when blood counts are low

10. Surgical interventions

a. No approved surgical interventions for leukemia exist

b. Bone marrow transplant is currently under investigation as a primary treatment for AML, ALL and CLL

11. Nursing interventions for patients undergoing surgery

a. Assist with pretransplant procedures, such as high-dose chemotherapy and total body irradiation, as appropriate

b. Teach the patient and family about bone marrow transplant procedures, including harvesting bone marrow from the donor and infusing harvested marrow into the patient

12. Radiotherapeutic interventions

a. Radiation therapy (RT) does not play a major role in treating leukemia

b. RT to the skull and spine may be used in maintenance therapy for ALL

c. RT to the spleen may be used to treat CML and ALL

d. Total body irradiation may be used to induce remission in CLL

e. Local RT to specific body sites may be used to treat CLL

f. Extracorporeal blood irradiation also may be used to reduce lymphocyte counts in CLL

g. RT may be used to ablate bone marrow before bone marrow transplant

13. Nursing interventions for patients receiving RT

a. Provide general nursing care measures applicable to all patients receiving RT (see Section II.C)

b. Teach the patient and family about the type of radiation to be used

14. Chemotherapeutic interventions

a. Chemotherapy is the primary treatment modality for leukemia

b. Chemotherapy seeks to reduce or eradicate the population of leukemic cells and promote repopulation of the bone marrow with normal cells

c. Success of chemotherapy depends on the type of leukemia, disease stage, availability of treatment resources, and the patient's overall health status

15. Chemotherapy in AML

a. The overriding goal of chemotherapy in AML is to eradicate disease. Treatment is considered successful if less than 5% of myeloblasts in the bone marrow

b. Chemotherapy in AML consists of four phases: induction, consolidation, maintenance, and reintensification

c. *Induction therapy* involves combination chemotherapy, using the cell cycle-specific antimetabolite cytosine arabinoside and an anthracycline agent, to induce severe bone marrow hypoplasia

d. Induction therapy drugs are given in a cycle over a few days; this cycle may be repeated if the initial cycle does not induce remission

e. *Consolidation therapy* is used when complete remission has been achieved

     f. Induction and consolidation may take up to 2 months, during which time support of the patient's bone marrow function is critical

     g. *Maintenance therapy* seeks to prevent recurrence of leukemic stem cells

     h. In maintenance therapy, different drugs and dosages are used to prevent the patient from developing a resistance to chemotherapeutic agents

     i. The patient may be able to resume normal activities during maintenance therapy

     j. The median duration of complete remission is 1 year

16. Chemotherapy in ALL

     a. The overriding goal of chemotherapy in ALL is to eradicate disease. Treatment is considered successful if it results in less than 5% of lymphoblasts in the bone marrow

     b. Agents used are selectively toxic to lymphoid tissues. Other hematopoietic cell lines are spared, resulting in decreased risk of toxicity and better tolerance to treatment

     c. Cell cycle-specific antimetabolites 6-mercaptopurine and methotrexate are used in combination with vincristine and prednisone to achieve a synergistic effect during induction therapy

     d. Support of the patient's bone marrow function is critical during severe bone marrow hypoplasia

     e. Maintenance therapy may involve systemic chemotherapy and prophylactic intrathecal chemotherapy

17. Chemotherapy in CML

     a. The goal of chemotherapy in CML is to induce reversion to the chronic asymptomatic state; complete remission (which would involve eradication of the Ph[1] chromosome) is impossible

     b. Initial therapy involves administering high doses of a fast-acting cytotoxic agent—such as busulfan, melphalan, or hydroxyurea—to decrease high WBC counts, often followed by a lower daily dose to maintain WBC counts within normal limits

     c. In some treatment centers, protocol calls for adminstering lower daily doses of these drugs only when the WBC count rises again

     d. Although relapses can be treated successfully, gradual resistance to therapy, myelofibrosis, or blast crisis may develop

     e. Treatment of blast crisis in CML is similar to treatment for AML or ALL; however, myeloblasts in CML are less responsive to treatment

18. Chemotherapy in CLL

     a. Chemotherapy in CLL seeks to palliate or prevent symptoms. Cure is not possible even with treatment, and the disease has a long course of progression even without treatment

     b. Chemotherapy usually is indicated for symptoms of anemia or lymphadenopathy

     c. Daily low doses of chlorambucil and prednisone may be given to decrease WBC counts

     d. In CLL, lymphocyte function may be abnormal despite normal WBC counts, which increases the risk of infection

e. Hypogammaglobulinemia and granulocytopenia also increase the risk of bacterial and fungal infection

19. Nursing interventions for patients receiving chemotherapy
    a. Provide general nursing care measures applicable to all patients receiving chemotherapy (see Section II.D)
    b. Assess for pain, ruptured blood vessels, increased intracranial pressure, and respiratory distress secondary to leukostasis
    c. Assess for petechiae, ecchymoses, and other signs and symptoms of bleeding secondary to thrombocytopenia or disseminated intravascular cogulation (DIC)
    d. Assess for early satiety, abdominal fullness, and abdominal pain or masses secondary to splenomegaly
    e. Monitor CBC for pancytopenia, secondary to treatment or hypersplenism
    f. Assess for joint pain and signs and symptoms of renal failure secondary to hyperuricemia
    g. If hyperuricemia develops, provide rigorous hydration, drug therapy with allopurinol, and dietary modifications, as ordered, to alkalinize urine
    h. Assess for early signs and symptoms of infection, which may develop if the patient is neutropenic, immunosuppressed, or taking steroids
    i. Administer antibiotics for prophylaxis or treatment, as ordered
    j. Administer blood products for anemia and thrombocytopenia, as ordered

C. Lymphomas: Hodgkin's disease
1. General information
   a. In Hodgkin's disease (HD), microscopic tissue examination reveals a multinucleated Reed-Steinberg giant cell
   b. HD is classified according to predominant cell type as nodular sclerosis, lymphocyte predominant, mixed cellular, or lymphocyte depleted
2. Epidemiology
   a. Each year in the United States, about 7,400 new cases of HD are diagnosed and 1,500 deaths occur from HD
   b. Incidence is about 33% higher in men than in women
   c. Incidence peaks between ages 20 and 30 and again between ages 60 and 70
   d. HD is more common in middle-class families and in developed countries
3. Risk factors
   a. Advanced socioeconomic status—higher social class, advanced education, small family size, and other factors that diminish or delay exposure to infectious agents and thus reduce immunity (in persons ages 20 to 30)
   b. Long-term occupational exposure to wood dust
   c. History of exposure to Epstein-Barr virus
4. Clinical manifestations
   a. Enlarged, painless, firm but rubbery, mobile lymph nodes
   b. Generalized lymphadenopathy
   c. Fever
   d. Night sweats
   e. Splenomegaly

   f. Weakness
   g. Fatigue
   h. Malaise
   i. Unexplained weight loss
   j. Malabsorption (with infiltration of small intestine by malignant lymphoma cells)
 5. Diagnostic tests
   a. CBC
   b. Erythrocyte sedimentation rate (ESR)
   c. Biopsy of involved lymph node or tissue
   d. Chest X-ray
   e. CT scan
 6. Staging
   a. The Ann Arbor modification of the Rye staging system for lymphoma is commonly used to stage HD
   b. Procedures used in staging include CBC; blood chemistries, including renal and liver function tests; liver-spleen scan; gallium scan; bone marrow biopsy; liver biopsy (if indicated by enlarged liver or abnormal liver function tests or scan); bilateral lymphangiography (if indicated by enlarged lymph nodes); staging laparotomy with multiple lymph node biopsies, splenectomy, liver and bone biopsy in specific situations
 7. Natural progression of disease
   a. Metastasis occurs primarily through orderly lymphatic spread; hematogenous spread also may occur
   b. Sites of metastasis include cervical, axillary, and inguinal lymph nodes; mediastinum; thymus gland; lungs and pleurae; heart and pericardium; spleen; liver; retroperitoneal and mesenteric lymph nodes; bone marrow; GI tract; and extranodal spread to the thyroid, skin, and kidneys
   c. Prognosis is based on disease stage and histologic cell type; 5-year survival rate ranges from 90% in lymphocyte predominant HD to 40% in mixed cellular and lymphocyte depleted HD
 8. Nursing interventions for screening, detection, and prevention
   a. Keep in mind that no screening tests for HD exist
   b. Be aware of the risk factors and signs and symptoms associated with HD
   c. Encourage and help a patient with possible signs and symptoms of HD to seek prompt medical attention
 9. Nursing interventions for psychosocial needs
   a. Encourage the patient to express feelings about the diagnosis, treatment plan, and impact of the disease on his life-style
   b. Assess patient and family coping mechanisms
   c. Determine the availability of support resources and help the patient gain access to appropriate resources
   d. Discuss the possible adverse effects of treatment
 10. Surgical interventions
   a. No routine surgical interventions exist for HD
   b. Surgery for HD is used primarily for diagnosis and staging

IRRADIATION PORTS

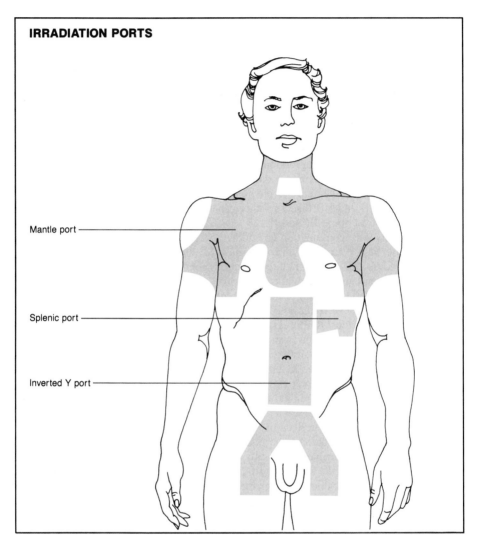

Mantle port

Splenic port

Inverted Y port

11. Nursing interventions for patients undergoing surgery for HD are similar to those for any patient undergoing surgery (see Section II.B)
12. Radiotherapeutic interventions
    a. RT is used to treat Stage I, Stage II, and Stage IIIA HD
    b. Total nodal irradiation ports may be used to radiate all major lymph node chains affected by HD
    c. Irradiation ports include the mantle port, inverted Y-port, and splenic port

13. Nursing interventions for patients receiving RT
   a. Provide general nursing care measures applicable to all patients receiving RT (see Section II.C)
   b. Inform a male patient and family that RT may cause temporary aspermia, but that proper shielding should preserve testicular function and spermatogenesis should resume after completion of treatment
   c. Explain to a female patient and family how oophoropexy before RT may preserve ovarian function
   d. Point out that RT may induce menopause unless ovarian shielding is used or oophoropexy is performed
14. Chemotherapeutic interventions
   a. Chemotherapy often is indicated in Stage IIIB and IV disease
   b. Some cancer centers use chemotherapy as an adjuvant to RT in treating Stage IB and IIB disease; other centers use chemotherapy only after relapse in Stage IB and IIB
   c. Trials with combination chemotherapy and radiotherapy are underway
   d. The MOPP regimen (nitrogen mustard, vincristine, procarbazine, prednisone) or ABVD (adriamycin, bleomycin, vinblastine, DTIC) regimen can effect remission in 80% of patients
   e. The ABVD regimen can effect remissions in about 50% of patients who fail to achieve remission with the MOPP regimen
   f. Likewise, the MOPP regimen may be used in an attempt to effect complete remissions in patients who fail to achieve remission with ABVD; response rate is lower, however
   g. Maintenance chemotherapy does not improve survival rate and thus is not indicated for treating HD
15. Nursing interventions for patients receiving chemotherapy
   a. Provide general nursing care measures applicable to all patients receiving chemotherapy (see Section II.D)
   b. Inform a male patient and family that the MOPP regimen may cause transient or permanent sterility
   c. Inform a female patient and family that the MOPP regimen may cause ovarian dysfunction but usually does not interfere with the ability to bear children
   d. Explain to male and female patients that the ABVD regimen causes less severe gonadal dysfunction than the MOPP regimen
   e. Instruct the patient and his or her partner in the use of birth control methods to prevent pregnancy during treatment periods

D. Lymphomas: Non-Hodgkin's lymphoma
1. General information
   a. In contrast to HD, Non-Hodgkin's lymphoma (NHL) is not associated with a Reed-Steinberg giant cell
   b. NHL is classified as well differentiated, poorly differentiated, mixed cell, histiocytic, undifferentiated, or unclassified

2. Epidemiology
   a. Each year in the United States about 31,700 new cases of NHL are diagnosed and 16,500 persons die from NHL
   b. Incidence of NHL is about 67% higher in men than in women
   c. Incidence increases starting between ages 40 and 50
3. Risk factors
   a. History of exposure to the Epstein-Barr virus (especially for Burkett's lymphoma)
   b. Immunodeficiency states, such as ataxia-telangiectasia and acquired immunodeficiency syndrome (AIDS)
   c. History of exposure to certain medications, including immunosuppressive and anticonvulsant drugs
4. Clinical manifestations
   a. Enlarged, painless, firm but rubbery, mobile lymph nodes
   b. Generalized lymphadenopathy
   c. Fever
   d. Night sweats
   e. Splenomegaly
   f. Weakness
   g. Fatigue
   h. Malaise
   i. Unexplained weight loss
   j. Gastric upset (with infiltration of the GI tract by malignant lymphomatous cells)
   k. Bone tumors
5. Diagnostic tests
   a. CBC
   b. ESR
   c. Biopsy of involved lymph node or tissue
   d. Chest X-ray
   e. CT scan
6. Staging
   a. The Ann Arbor modification of the Rye staging system for lymphoma is used to stage NHL
   b. Procedures used in staging include CBC, blood chemistries, liver-spleen scan, bone marrow biopsy, liver biopsy (if indicated by enlarged spleen or abnormal liver function tests or scans), and bilateral lymphangiography (if indicated by enlarged lymph nodes)
7. Natural progression of disease
   a. Routes of metastasis include lymphatic spread and hematogenous spread
   b. Sites of metastasis include cervical, axillary, and inguinal lymph nodes; mediastinum; thymus gland; lungs and pleurae; heart and pericardium; spleen; liver; retroperitoneal and mesenteric lymph nodes; bone marrow; GI tract; and extranodal spread to the thyroid, skin, and kidneys
   c. Prognosis is based on histologic cell type; 3-year survival rate ranges from 100% for well differentiated to 25% for histiocytic lymphoma

8. Nursing interventions for screening, detection, and prevention
   a. Keep in mind that no screening tests for NHL exist
   b. Be aware of the risk factors and signs and symptoms associated with NHL
   c. Encourage a patient with possible signs and symptoms of NHL to seek prompt medical attention
9. Nursing interventions for psychosocial needs
   a. Encourage the patient to express feelings about the diagnosis, treatment plan, and impact of the disease on his life-style
   b. Assess patient and family coping mechanisms
   c. Determine the availability of support resources and help the patient gain access to appropriate resources
10. Surgical interventions
    a. No routine surgical interventions exist for NHL
    b. Surgery is used primarily for diagnosis
11. Nursing interventions for patients undergoing surgery for NHL are similar to those for any patient undergoing surgery (see Section II.B)
12. Radiotherapeutic interventions
    a. RT is rarely used to treat NHL because of the disease's wide variety of cell types and diffuse nature
    b. RT may be used in early-stage NHL when all disease sites can be irradiated
    c. Total nodal irradiation is rarely used in NHL
    d. RT may be used to palliate symptomatic areas unresponsive to chemotherapy
13. Nursing interventions for patients receiving RT
    a. Provide general nursing care measures applicable to all patients receiving RT (see Section II.C)
    b. Assess for adverse effects during and after treatment
    c. Provide support and guidance during periods of remission
14. Chemotherapeutic interventions
    a. Chemotherapy is the preferred treatment for Stage III, Stage IV, and some Stage II disease
    b. Intensive combination chemotherapy is used for aggressive, diffuse NHL; one possible combination consists of an alkylating agent, a vinca alkaloid, a glucocorticoid, and an antibiotic antineoplastic agent such as bleomycin or doxorubicin
    c. Combination chemotherapy also has been used for less aggressive nodular NHL. Some experts advocate palliating symptoms by using RT on symptomatic areas, followed by chemotherapy as the disease becomes more aggressive
15. Nursing interventions for patients receiving chemotherapy
    a. Provide general nursing care measures applicable to all patients receiving chemotherapy (see Section II.D)
    b. Be aware that cumulative drug toxicity may occur; monitor for signs and symptoms of toxicity

Points to Remember

Leukemia is classified according to the stage at which cellular maturation stops.

Leukemic cells crowd out normal bone marrow cells and inhibit normal cell growth and function.

Hodgkin's disease (HD) spreads through the lymphatic system in an orderly fashion.

In HD, a Reed-Steinberg giant cell is present on microscopic examination of tissues.

Non-Hodgkin's lymphoma (NHL) often is widespread by the time of diagnosis.

Chemotherapy is the primary treatment modality for leukemia and NHL; RT and chemotherapy are used to treat HD.

Glossary

Bone marrow aspiration—procedure to remove bone marrow using a suction technique

Mantle RT—irradiation of the cervical, supraclavicular, axillary, and mediastinal lymph nodes (so called because it irradiates an area that would be covered by a mantle or cloak)

Oophoropexy—surgical suspension of an ovary to the abdominal wall

Pancytopenia—abnormal condition characterized by a marked reduction in erythrocytes, leukocytes, and platelets

Sanctuary sites—body areas into which cytotoxic drugs cannot permeate and where cancer cells can escape the tumorcidal effects of chemotherapy

Oncologic Emergencies

Learning Objectives

After studying this section, the reader should be able to:

- Identify selected oncologic emergencies.

- Discuss general characteristics of each of these emergencies.

- Identify possible diagnostic test findings associated with each emergency.

- Describe possible patient assessment findings associated with each emergency.

- Identify possible nursing interventions in each emergency.

XIII. Oncologic Emergencies

A. Introduction
1. Oncologic emergencies are life-threatening conditions requiring prompt medical treatment
2. Such conditions may result from
   a. Tumor or tumor byproducts
   b. Secondary involvement or other organs by malignant disease spread
   c. Adverse effects of cancer treatment

B. Cardiac tamponade
1. General information
   a. In cardiac tamponade, fluid accumulation and increased pressure in the pericaridal sac inhibits ventricular expansion and heart filling, resulting in impaired heart function
   b. Mechanisms normally regulating cardiac output eventually fail to compensate for increased intrapericardial pressure, and total circulatory collapse may result
   c. Fluid accumulation from tumor presence or pericardial thickening secondary to radiation therapy may cause increased intrapericardial pressure
   d. Cancers most likely to affect the pericardium include breast cancer, leukemia, melanomas, and lymphomas
   e. The primary goal of treatment is maintaining adequate cardiac and pulmonary function
2. Diagnostic test findings
   a. Chest X-ray: cardiomegaly, pericardial thickening or effusion
   b. Echocardiogram: pericardial effusion or thickening, abnormal cardiac motion
   c. ECG: sinus tachycardia, dysrhythmias, elevated ST segment, various T-wave changes
   d. Pericardial fluid cytology: presence of serosanguinous fluid
3. Assessment findings
   a. Severe dyspnea
   b. Cough
   c. Cyanosis
   d. Extreme anxiety and apprehension
   e. Narrowed pulse pressure
   f. Paradoxical pulse
   g. Tachycardia
   h. Dysrhythmias
   i. Faint heart sounds
   j. Elevated central venous pressure
   k. Altered level of consciousness (LOC)
   l. Pericardial friction rub
   m. Pale, ashen, diaphoretic skin
   n. Hepatomegaly

4. Nursing interventions
   a. Maintain the patient on bed rest and minimal activity to decrease oxygen demand
   b. Elevate the head of the bed 30 to 45 degrees to promote adequate oxygenation
   c. Administer oxygen, as ordered, to prevent hypoxia
   d. Administer medications to relieve anxiety and pain, as ordered
   e. Assess cardiopulmonary status by checking vital signs, pulses, ECG readings, and heart sounds for abnormalities
   f. Monitor arterial pressure readings to detect changes in hemodynamic status
   g. Monitor laboratory values, such as arterial blood gases (ABG), complete blood count (CBC), and serum electrolytes, for abnormalities
   h. Assess fluid volume status—e.g., amount of peripheral edema, intake and output, and body weight fluctuations—to detect fluid imbalance
   i. Administer I.V. fluids, as ordered, to maintain intravascular volume and perfusion
   j. Administer vasopressors, cardiac medications, and diuretics, as ordered, to maintain intravascular perfusion and volume
   k. Provide emotional support to the patient and family and encourage them to express their fears and concerns

C. Superior vena cava syndrome
1. General information
   a. Superior vena cava syndrome (SVCS) involves impaired venous return from the head, upper thorax, and arms caused by occlusion of the superior vena cava
   b. Cancers commonly associated with SVCS include lung cancer, lymphomas, and breast cancer
2. Diagnostic test findings: chest X-ray indicating mediastinal or lung mass
3. Assessment findings
   a. Facial and periorbital edema
   b. Venous distention in the neck and upper thorax
   c. Edema of the neck, upper thorax, and arms
   d. Conjunctival and retinal vein edema
   e. Dyspnea
   f. Headache
   g. Chest pain
   h. Dysphagia
   i. Cough
   j. Tachycardia
   k. Tachypnea
   l. Horner's syndrome: eyelid droop, pupil constriction, and conjunctivitis in one eye, and anhidrosis (absence of sweat) on one side of the face
   m. Visual disturbances
   n. Hoarseness

    o. Severe upper airway obstruction
    p. Altered LOC
4. Nursing interventions
    a. Assess cardiopulmonary status for abnormalities, such as abnormal heart or lung sounds
    b. Elevate head of bed 30 to 45 degrees to ease breathing
    c. Administer oxygen, as ordered, to prevent hypoxia
    d. Monitor vital signs for changes
    e. Assess LOC and reorient if necessary
    f. Monitor presence and amount of facial and periorbital edema
    g. Monitor intake and output to prevent fluid imbalance
    h. Assess ability to talk, eat, and drink, and report any changes
    i. Assess for headache and chest pain
    j. Administer medications to relieve pain and anxiety, as ordered
    k. Provide safety measures as needed to prevent injury

D. Hypercalcemia
1. General information
    a. Hypercalcemia, defined as a serum calcium concentration >11 mg/dl, occurs when calcium enters serum more rapidly than it is removed
    b. Multiple myeloma causes approximately 50% of cancer-related hypercalcemia
    c. Other metastatic cancers associated with hypercalcemia include breast cancer, lung cancer, and renal cancer
2. Diagnostic test findings
    a. Serum calcium: >11 mg/dl
    b. Urinary calcium: increased
    c. Blood urea nitrogen and creatinine: increased
    d. Serum phosphate: increased
    e. Serum potassium: decreased
    f. ECG: prolonged P-R interval, widened T-wave, shortened Q-T interval, or prolonged Q-T interval (with serum calcium level >16 mg/dl)
3. Assessment findings
    a. Polyuria
    b. Dehydration
    c. Polydipsia
    d. Constipation
    e. Fatigue
    f. Muscle weakness
    g. Diminished deep tendon reflexes
    h. Anorexia
    i. Nausea and vomiting
    j. Dysrhythmias
    k. Paralytic ileus
    l. Bone pain
    m. Altered LOC progressing to stupor and coma

4. Nursing interventions
   a. Teach the patient and family about the signs and symtpoms of hypercalcemia and possible treatment measures
   b. Promote ambulation and exercise to prevent excessive calcium loss resulting from immobility
   c. Maintain fluid intake up to 3 liters/day to ensure adequate elimination of calcium
   d. Monitor intake and output and intervene as necessary to maintain fluid balance
   e. Evaluate blood chemistries—especially serum calcium and phosphate levels— for significant changes
   f. Assess vital signs for abnormalities
   g. Monitor ECG readings and administer antiarrhythmics, as ordered
   h. Assess LOC and report any significant changes
   i. Anticipate changes in LOC and provide safety measures as necessary to prevent patient injury
   j. Assess GI tract function
   k. Assess for complaints of nausea, vomiting, or excessive thirst; administer antiemetics, as ordered
   l. Assess deep tendon reflexes
   m. Administer analgesics as necessary to relieve pain
   n. Teach the patient and family about the role of a low-calcium diet in preventing hypercalcemia

E. Sepsis
   1. General information
      a. Sepsis refers to the presence of pathogenic organisms or endotoxins in blood or other tissues, and to conditions resulting from such presence
      b. Sepsis most commonly results from gram-negative bacteria. It also may result from fungal or viral infection or parasites
      c. Sepsis is the leading cause of death in patients with treatment-induced neutropenia
   2. Diagnostic test findings
      a. Blood cultures: positive organism growth
      b. CBC: increased white blood cell count (possibly decreased in immunocompromised patients)
      c. ABG: metabolic acidosis
      d. Prothrombin time (PT) and partial thromboplastin time (PTT): prolonged clotting times
      e. Chest X-ray: presence of infiltrate
   3. Assessment findings
      a. Temperature above 102° F. (39° C.)
      b. Chills
      c. Flushed, warm dry skin
      d. Widened pulse pressure
      e. Decreased blood pressure

      f. Anxiety

      g. Confusion

      h. Lethargy

   4. Nursing interventions

      a. Encourage frequent hand washing to prevent transmission of organisms

      b. Use aseptic technique during invasive procedures to prevent contamination

      c. Check areas of broken skin for signs of infection

      d. Assess vital signs—especially temperature and pulse—for changes that may indicate infection

      e. Assess for signs and symptoms of septic shock

      f. Assess lung sounds for abnormalities that may point to pneumonia

      g. Assess for signs and symptoms of bleeding, especially if PT and PTT are abnormal

      h. Monitor LOC and report any significant changes

      i. Institute safety precautions to prevent patient injury

      j. Assess hemodynamic status and administer I.V. fluid volume replacements as ordered to maintain hemodynamic status and prevent circulatory collapse

      k. Provide neutropenic precautions as necessary and according to institutional policy

      l. Administer antibiotics, as ordered, to control infection

     m. Evaluate results of laboratory tests, such as blood cultures and CBC, for significant changes

      n. Explain all aspects of treatment, including the reasons for certain interventions, to the patient and family

F. Spinal cord compression

   1. General information

      a. Spinal cord compression involves pressure on the spinal cord that results in partial or total loss of nerve function and possibly vertebral collapse

      b. It often is caused by tumor invasion into the spinal canal. Primary tumors that metastasize to bone are the most common cause; these include lung cancer, breast cancer, kidney cancer, melanomas, GI tract tumors, prostatic cancer, and cervical cancer

      c. Spinal cord damage may result either directly from tumor invasion or indirectly from ischemia caused by cord compression

   2. Diagnostic test findings

      a. Spinal X-rays: spinal erosion, spinal calcification

      b. Myelography: presence of tumor mass, compression

      c. Lumbar puncture: changes in color and composition of cerebrospinal fluid

   3. Assessment findings

      a. Localized back pain or pain referred from the involved nerve root

      b. Motor deficits, such as muscle weakness and hypotonicity, ataxia, and hyporeflexia

    c. Sensory deficits, such as numbness, paresthesias, loss of temperature sensation, paraplegia, and urine or fecal incontinence or retention

    d. Spinal shock involving the loss of motor, sensory, autonomic, and reflex function below the level of involvement (severity and duration is related to the speed of progression and success in relieving compression)

    e. Respiratory arrest (with involvement of cervical vertebrae C1 to C3)

4. Nursing interventions

    a. Assess neurologic status, including sensory and motor function, LOC, and level of pain

    b. Assess bowel and bladder function for incontinence or retention; as necessary, assist with measures to control bladder and bowel function

    c. Assist with traction application if ordered

    d. Maintain the patient on bed rest, if needed

    e. Assess for proper body alignment and intervene as necessary to prevent contractures

    f. Provide meticulous skin care to prevent skin breakdown

    g. Encourage the patient to perform range-of-motion exercises to maintain and improve mobility; assist as necessary

    h. Use the log-roll technique when turning or transferring the patient to prevent spinal flexion

    i. Encourage the patient to turn, cough, and deep-breathe often to prevent atelectasis resulting from immobility

    j. Assist the patient with activities of daily living as needed

    k. Provide safety measures to prevent patient injury

    l. Administer analgesics for pain relief as needed

    m. Explain all aspects of treatment, along with the reasons for the treatments, to the patient and family

    n. Involve the patient and family in the plan of care

    o. Promote early rehabilitation to return the patient to an optimum level of function

G. Syndrome of inappropriate antidiuretic hormone

1. General information

    a. Syndrome of inappropriate antidiuretic hormone (SIADH) results from excessive release of antidiuretic hormone (ADH) and is characterized by extracellular hypo-osmolality, water intoxication, hyponatremia, normovolemia, hypertonic urine, and normal renal and adrenal function

    b. It is associated with oat cell and other bronchogenic cancers, pancreatic cancer, prostatic cancer, Hodgkin's disease, and administration of high-dose cyclophosphamide therapy

    c. Symptoms develop when serum sodium levels drop below 120mEq/l

2. Diagnostic test findings

    a. Serum sodium: <130mEq/l

    b. Serum osmolality: <280 mOsm/kg

    c. Urine osmolality: <500 mOsm/kg

    d. Urine sodium: >20mEq/l

     e. Serum potassium: decreased

     f. Serum calcium: decreased

     g. Blood urea nitrogen and creatinine: decreased

3. Assessment findings

     a. Weight gain

     b. Edema

     c. Fatigue

     d. Weakness

     e. Lethargy

     f. Headache

     g. Confusion

     h. Irritability

     i. Anorexia

     j. Nausea and vomiting

     k. Diarrhea

     l. Muscle cramps

     m. Hyporeflexia

     n. Convulsions

4. Nursing interventions

     a. Assess for signs and symptoms of SIADH in high-risk patients

     b. Monitor serum and urinary sodium levels

     c. Assess fluid balance, carefully monitor intake and output, weigh patient daily, and maintain fluid restrictions as ordered

     d. Assess lung sounds for abnormalities that may indicate fluid accumulation

     e. Monitor urine specific gravity to detect hypertonicity

     f. Monitor vital signs for abnormalities

     g. Assess neurologic status, watching particularly for altered LOC, and reorient the patient as necessary

     h. Provide safety measures as necessary to prevent patient injury

     i. Keep in mind that a patient with SIADH may require reduced dosages of certain medications, such as procainamide, morphine, chlorpropamide, and digoxin

     j. Explain all aspects of treatment and the reasons for each intervention to the patient and family

H. Tumor lysis syndrome

1. General information

     a. Tumor lysis syndrome is a metabolic imbalance characterized by hyperuricemia, hyperkalemia, hyperphosphatemia, and hypocalcemia

     b. This syndrome is caused by rapid cell destruction and turnover resulting from chemotherapy; it usually develops within 5 days after start of chemotherapy

     c. Cancers commonly associated with tumor lysis syndrome include non-Hodgkin's lymphoma, acute lymphoblastic leukemia, and chronic leukemia in the blast phase

2. Diagnostic test findings
   a. Serum potassium: increased
   b. Serum phosphate: increased
   c. Serum uric acid: increased
   d. Serum calcium: decreased
   e. Blood urea nitrogen and creatinine: increased
   f. Lactic dehydrogenase: increased
3. Assessment findings (depend on the predominant chemical imbalance)
   a. Bradycardia
   b. Heart block
   c. Ventricular dysrhythmias
   d. Cardiac arrest
   e. Weakness
   f. Lethargy
   g. Muscle twitching and cramping
   h. Paresthesias
   i. Confusion
   j. Tetany
   k. Convulsions
   l. Oliguria
   m. Renal insufficiency and failure
4. Nursing interventions
   a. Keep in mind that the most effective intervention is prevention or early detection of tumor lysis syndrome
   b. Assess for signs and symptoms of tumor lysis syndrome in high-risk patients
   c. Make sure that patients receive allopurinol before chemotherapy begins, in order to reduce uric acid concentration
   d. Explain the purpose of allopurinol administration to the patient and family
   e. Maintain adequate hydration during chemotherapy to help ensure adequate renal function
   f. Assess laboratory data, such as serum electrolytes, and intervene as necessary to prevent imbalances
   g. Teach the patient and family about dietary modifications to increase urine alkalinity
   h. Administer calcium supplements, as ordered, to prevent hypocalcemia
   i. Monitor ECG readings for changes that may indicate metabolic imbalance
   j. Prepare the patient for hemodialysis if renal failure occurs

I. Disseminated intravascular coagulation
1. General information
   a. Disseminated intravascular coagulation (DIC) involves an abnormal activation of both coagulation and fibrinolytic factors, leading to uncontrolled bleeding and thrombus formation

      b. Cancers commonly associated with DIC include lung cancer, prostatic cancer, and leukemia

2. Diagnostic test findings
   a. Prothrombin time: prolonged
   b. Partial thromboplastin time: prolonged
   c. Platelet count: <150,000/mm³
   d. Fibrinogen level: <150 mg/dl
   e. Fibrin degradation products: increased
3. Assessment findings
   a. Petechiae
   b. Ecchymoses
   c. Cyanosis
   d. Epistaxis
   e. Conjunctival bleeding
   f. Hematemesis
   g. Frank or occult blood in stools
   h. Hematuria
   i. Menorrhagia or metrorrhagia
   j. Oliguria or anuria
   k. Hemoptysis
   l. Dyspnea
   m. Restlessness
   n. Altered LOC
   o. Tachycardia
   p. Cold, moist skin
4. Nursing interventions
   a. Monitor cardiopulmonary status for changes indicating blood loss
   b. Monitor coagulation studies for abnormalities
   c. Assess body orifices for frank bleeding
   d. Accurately record and report any blood loss
   e. Institute bleeding precautions—such as avoiding trauma, venipunctures, and intramuscular injections—to prevent complications from bleeding
   f. Perform oral care with cotton-tipped applicators and a toothette to prevent bleeding
   g. Encourage the patient to avoid medications which interfere with platelet function—such as products containing aspirin, which may prolong bleeding time
   h. Watch for early signs and symptoms of DIC, such as venous induration and distention, muscle tenderness, fever, and chills
   i. Administer I.V. fluids, as ordered, to maintain adequate fluid volume
   j. Administer anticoagulant therapy, as ordered, to inhibit further clot formation
   k. Encourage the patient to avoid leg-crossing to prevent venous stasis
   l. Provide pain control measures, including administering analgesics, as ordered
   m. Promote adequate circulation to patient's extremities to prevent thrombus formation

Points to Remember

Oncologic emergencies can be life-threatening and require prompt attention.

Timely, accurate assessment and intervention by the nurse and other multidisciplinary health care team members can help prevent or minimize problems.

Maintaining adequate cardiac and pulmonary function is essential during any oncologic emergency.

Glossary

Ataxia—abnormal condition marked by impaired ability to coordinate movements

Endotoxin—toxin found in the cell walls of some bacteria (especially gram-negative bacteria) that is released when the bacteria dies and is broken down by the body

Ischemia—insufficient blood supply to a body part resulting from vascular constriction or obstruction

Index

A

Acral-lentiginous melanomas, 64
Acute lymphoblastic leukemia, 137
  chemotherapy in, 140
Acute myelogenous leukemia, 135
  chemotherapy in, 139-140
Alkylating agents, 28
Alopecia, management of, 40-41
Anaplasia, 6
Anemia, management of, 41-42
Antimetabolites, 29-30
Antineoplastic agents, 26-31
  cell cycle and, 27i
Antineoplastic antibiotics, 29

B

Basal cell carcinoma, 66-68
Bereavement, 60-61
Bladder cancer, 104-107
  interventions for, 105-107
  risk factors for, 104
  staging of, 105
Blood cell differentiation, 136i
Breast cancer, 117-121
  interventions for, 119-121
  risk factors for, 118
  staging of, 118
Bronchogenic cancer, 75-78
  interventions for, 76-78
  risk factors for, 75-76
  staging of, 76

C

Cachexia, 39
Cancer therapy, principles of, 13-24
Carcinogenesis, theories of, 9
Cardiac tamponade as oncologic emergency, 149-150
Cervical cancer, 121-125
  interventions for, 123-125
  risk factors for, 122
  staging of, 123
Chemotherapy
  adverse effects of, 21
  equipment used to administer, 21
  extravasation of antineoplastic agents and, 22
  goals of, 20
  mechanisms of action of, 21
  nursing interventions for patients receiving, 22-23
  principle for, 20
  routes of administration for, 21
  safety guidelines for, 21-22
Chronic lymphocytic leukemia, 137
  chemotherapy in, 140-141
Chronic myelogenous leukemia, 137
  chemotherapy in, 140
Colorectal cancer, 94-98
  interventions for, 96-98
  risk factors for, 95
  staging of, 96

Constipation, management of, 43-44
Coping ability, patient's, 54-59
Curative surgery, 14

D

Diagnostic surgery, 14
Diarrhea, management of, 44-45
Disseminated intravascular coagulation as oncologic
  emergency, 156-157
Dysplasia, 6

E

En bloc resection, 24
Endometrial cancer, 125-128
  interventions for, 127-128
  risk factors for, 126
  staging of, 126
Esophageal cancer, 81-85
  interventions for, 82-85
  risk factors for, 81
  staging of, 82

FG

Fatigue, management of, 45-46
Gastric cancer, 85-87
  interventions for, 86-88
  risk factors for, 86
  staging of, 86
Gastrointestinal tract, cancer of the, 81-99
Grief, 60

H

Head and neck cancer, 71-75
  interventions for, 72-75
  risk factors for, 71
  staging of, 72
Hematologic system, cancer of the, 135-147
Hodgkin's disease, 141-144
  interventions for, 142-144
  irradiation ports for, 143i
  risk factors for, 141
  staging, 142
Hormonal antineoplastic agents, 30-31
Hospice, 11
Hypercalcemia as oncologic emergency, 151-152
Hyperplasia, 6

IJKL

Immune system, function of, in cancer, 9-10
Invasion, 9
Lentigo maligna melanomas, 64
Leukemia, 135, 137-141
  interventions for, 138-141
  risk factors for, 137
Liver cancer, 91-94
  interventions for, 93-94
  risk factors for, 92
  staging of, 92

i refers to an illustration.

Lung cancer. *See* Bronchogenic cancer.
Lymphomas, 141-146

M

Malignant melanomas, 64-66
  interventions for, 65-66
  risk factors for, 64
  staging of, 65
Mechanical device insertion, 15
Metaplasia, 6
Metastasis, 9
Mucositis, management of, 49-50

N

Nausea, management of, 46
Neoplasm, 6
  classification of, 7
Neoplastic nomenclature, 7
Neutropenia, management of, 46-47
Nodular melanomas, 64
Non-Hodgkin's lymphoma, 144-146
  interventions for, 146
  risk factors for, 145
  staging of, 145
Nonmelanomas, 66-68
  interventions for, 67-68
  risk factors for, 67
  staging of, 67
Nutritional status
  assessment of, 36
  cancer-related causes of imbalance in, 34-35
  effects of cancer surgery on, 35
  effects of chemotherapy on, 35
  effects of radiation therapy on, 35
Nutritional support therapy
  enteral tube feedings, 37
  oral, 36
  peripheral parenteral, 37
  total parenteral, 37-38

O

Oncologic emergencies, 149-158
Ovarian cancer, 129-132
  interventions for, 130-132
  risk factors for, 129
  staging of, 129-130

PQ

Pain, management of, 47-49
Palliative surgery, 14
Pancreatic cancer, 88-91
  interventions for, 90-91
  risk factors for, 89
  staging of, 89
Prophylactic surgery, 14
Prostatic cancer, 110-114
  interventions for, 111-114
  risk factors for, 110
  staging of, 111
Psychosocial needs, family's, management of, 54-62
  in acute phase, 54-55
  in bereavement phase, 60-61
  in chronic phase, 56-58
  in terminal phase, 58-59

Psychosocial needs, patient's, management of, 54-59
  in acute phase, 54-55
  in chronic phase, 56-58
  in terminal phase, 58-59

R

Radiation therapy
  adverse effects of, 19
  factors affecting patient response to, 17-18
  goals of, 17
  mechanism of action of, 18-19
  nursing interventions for patients receiving, 20
  principle for, 17
  safety measures and, 19-20
  types of, 18
  types of radiation used in, 18
Reconstructive surgery, 15
Renal cancer, 101-103
  interventions for, 102-103
  risk factors for, 101
  staging of, 102
Reproductive tract, cancer of the, 110-133

S

Sanctuary sites, chemotherapy and, 147
Sepsis as oncologic emergency, 152-153
Skin cancer, 64-69
Spinal cord compression as oncologic emergency,
  153-154
Squamocolumnar junction, cervical cancer and, 122i
Squamous cell carcinoma, 66-68
Staging systems, 7
Stomatitis, management of, 49-50
Superficial spreading melanomas, 64
Superior vena cava syndrome as oncologic emergency,
  150-151
Surgery
  adverse effects of, 15
  factors affecting patient's response to, 14
  goals of, 13-14
  mechanism of action of, 15
  nursing interventions for patients undergoing, 15-17
  principles for, 13
  types of, 14-15
Syndrome of inappropriate antidiuretic hormone as oncologic emergency, 154-155

T

Testicular cancer, 114-117
  interventions for, 115-117
  risk factors for, 115
  staging of, 115
Thrombocytopenia, management of, 50-51
Treatment modalities, 6
Tumor, node, metastasis (TNM) staging system, 8
Tumor angiogenesis factor, 11
Tumor lysis syndrome as oncologic emergency, 156-156

U

Urinary tract, cancer of the, 101-108

VWXYZ

Vinca alkaloids, 31
Vomiting, management of, 46